ORTHOPEDIC CLINICS OF NORTH AMERICA

www.orthopedic.theclinics.com

Controversies in Fracture Care

January 2017 • Volume 48 • Number 1

Editors

FREDERICK M. AZAR
JAMES H. CALANDRUCCIO
BENJAMIN J. GREAR
BENJAMIN M. MAUCK
JEFFREY R. SAWYER
PATRICK C. TOY
JOHN C. WEINLEIN

ELSEVIER

1600 John F. Kennedy Boulevard • Suite 1800 • Philadelphia, Pennsylvania, 19103-2899.

http://www.orthopedic.theclinics.com

ORTHOPEDIC CLINICS OF NORTH AMERICA Volume 48, Number 1
January 2017 ISSN 0030-5898, ISBN-13: 978-0-323-48265-3

Editor: Lauren Boyle
Developmental Editor: Kristen Helm

Orthopedic Clinics of North America (ISSN 0030-5898) is published quarterly by Elsevier Inc., 360 Park Avenue South, New York, NY 10010-1710. Months of issue are January, April, July, and October. Business and Editorial Offices: 1600 John F. Kennedy Blvd., Suite 1800, Philadelphia, PA 19103-2899. Customer Service Office: 3251 Riverport Lane, Maryland Heights, MO 63043. Periodicals postage paid at New York, NY and additional mailing offices. Subscription prices are $319.00 per year for (US individuals), $686.00 per year for (US institutions), $376.00 per year (Canadian individuals), $837.00 per year (Canadian institutions), $464.00 per year (international individuals), $837.00 per year (international institutions), $100.00 per year (US students), $220.00 per year (Canadian and international students). Foreign air speed delivery is included in all *Clinics* subscription prices. All prices are subject to change without notice. **POSTMASTER: Send change of address to** *Orthopedic Clinics of North America*, **Elsevier Health Sciences Division, Subscription Customer Service, 3251 Riverport Lane, Maryland Heights, MO 63043. Customer Service (orders, claims, online, change of address): Elsevier Health Sciences Division, Subscription Customer Service, 3251 Riverport Lane, Maryland Heights, MO 63043. Tel: 1-800-654-2452 (U.S. and Canada); 314-447-8871 (outside U.S. and Canada). Fax: 314-447-8029. E-mail:** journalscustomerservice-usa@elsevier.com **(for print support);** journalsonlinesupport-usa@elsevier.com **(for online support).**

Reprints. For copies of 100 or more, of articles in this publication, please contact the Commercial Reprints Department, Elsevier Inc., 360 Park Avenue South, New York, NY 10010-1710. Tel.: 212-633-3874; Fax: 212-633-3820; E-mail: reprints@elsevier.com.

Orthopedic Clinics of North America is covered in *MEDLINE/PubMed (Index Medicus)*, *Cinahl, Excerpta Medica*, and *Cumulative Index to Nursing and Allied Health Literature*.

PROGRAM OBJECTIVE

Orthopedic Clinics of North America offers clinical review articles on the most cutting-edge technologies and techniques in the field, including adult reconstruction, the upper extremity, pediatrics, trauma, oncology, and sports medicine.

TARGET AUDIENCE

Practicing orthopedic surgeons, orthopedic residents, and other healthcare professionals who specialize in orthopedic technologies and techniques for adult reconstruction, the upper extremity, pediatrics, trauma, oncology, and sports medicine.

LEARNING OBJECTIVES

Upon completion of this activity, participants will be able to:
1. Review complications in pediatric fracture management.
2. Discuss current controversy in care of fractures including calcaneal fractures, ankle fractures, and malleolar fractures, and other fractures of the lower extremity.
3. Recognize controversy in the care of ulnar fractures, clavicular fractures, and other fractures of the upper extremity.

ACCREDITATION

The Elsevier Office of Continuing Medical Education (EOCME) is accredited by the Accreditation Council for Continuing Medical Education (ACCME) to provide continuing medical education for physicians.

The EOCME designates this enduring material for a maximum of 15 *AMA PRA Category 1 Credit*(s)™. Physicians should claim only the credit commensurate with the extent of their participation in the activity.

All other health care professionals requesting continuing education credit for this enduring material will be issued a certificate of participation.

DISCLOSURE OF CONFLICTS OF INTEREST

The EOCME assesses conflict of interest with its instructors, faculty, planners, and other individuals who are in a position to control the content of CME activities. All relevant conflicts of interest that are identified are thoroughly vetted by EOCME for fair balance, scientific objectivity, and patient care recommendations. EOCME is committed to providing its learners with CME activities that promote improvements or quality in healthcare and not a specific proprietary business or a commercial interest.

The planning committee, staff, authors and editors listed below have identified no financial relationships or relationships to products or devices they or their spouse/life partner have with commercial interest related to the content of this CME activity:

Lindsay Andras, MD; Frederick M. Azar, MD; William R. Barfield, PhD; Jason Bariteau, MD; Walter B. Beaver Jr, MD; Lauren Boyle; Nathan Bruck, MD; James H. Calandruccio, MD; Cara Cipriano, MD; Keith P. Connolly, MD; Brian Curtin, MD; Jaime R. Denning, MD; Nicholas Erdle, MD; Anjali Fortna; Heather E. Gotha, MD; Benjamin J. Grear, MD; Langdon A. Hartsock, MD; Robert E. Holmes, MD; Christopher M. Hopkins, MD; Kai Li, MD; Samir Mehta, MD; Jeffrey G. Mokris, MD; Premkumar Nandhakumar; Susan M. Odum, PhD; Joshua C. Rozell, MD; Nachshon Shazar, MD; Bryan D. Springer, MD; Louis S. Stryker, MD; Megan Suermann; Shay Tenenbaum, MD; Patrick C. Toy, MD; David N. Vegari, MD; Scott Yang, MD; Jacob R. Zide, MD.

The planning committee, staff, authors and editors listed below have identified financial relationships or relationships to products or devices they or their spouse/life partner have with commercial interest related to the content of this CME activity:

Thomas K. Fehring, MD is on the speakers' bureau for, is a consultant/advisor for, has research support from, and receives royalties/patents from, DePuy Synthes, a Johnson & Johnson Company.
Benjamin M. Mauck, MD is a consultant/advisor for Olympus America.
Jeffrey R. Sawyer, MD is on the speakers' bureau for and is a consultant/advisor for Johnson & Johnson Services, Inc, and receives royalties/patents from Elsevier.
John C. Weinlein, MD receives roylaties/patents from Elsevier.

UNAPPROVED/OFF-LABEL USE DISCLOSURE

The EOCME requires CME faculty to disclose to the participants:
1. When products or procedures being discussed are off-label, unlabelled, experimental, and/or investigational (not US Food and Drug Administration [FDA] approved); and
2. Any limitations on the information presented, such as data that are preliminary or that represent ongoing research, interim analyses, and/or unsupported opinions. Faculty may discuss information about pharmaceutical agents that is outside of FDA-approved labelling. This information is intended solely for CME and is not intended to promote off-label use of these medications. If you have any questions, contact the medical affairs department of the manufacturer for the most recent prescribing information.

TO ENROLL

To enroll in the *Orthopedic Clinics of North America* Continuing Medical Education program, call customer service at 1-800-654-2452 or sign up online at http://www.theclinics.com/home/cme. The CME program is available to subscribers for an additional annual fee of USD 215.

METHOD OF PARTICIPATION

In order to claim credit, participants must complete the following:

1. Complete enrolment as indicated above.
2. Read the activity.
3. Complete the CME Test and Evaluation. Participants must achieve a score of 70% on the test. All CME Tests and Evaluations must be completed online.

CME INQUIRIES/SPECIAL NEEDS

For all CME inquiries or special needs, please contact elsevierCME@elsevier.com.

EDITORIAL BOARD

CONTRIBUTORS

AUTHORS

LINDSAY ANDRAS, MD
Assistant Professor of Orthopaedic Surgery,
Children's Orthopaedic Center, Children's
Hospital Los Angeles, Los Angeles, California

WILLIAM R. BARFIELD, PhD
Department of Orthopaedics, Medical
University of South Carolina, Charleston,
South Carolina

JASON BARITEAU, MD
Assistant Professor of Orthopedics, Emory
University School of Medicine, Atlanta,
Georgia

WALTER B. BEAVER Jr, MD
Surgeon, OrthoCarolina Hip & Knee Center,
Charlotte, North Carolina

NATHAN BRUCK, MD
Department of Orthopedic Surgery, Chaim
Sheba Medical Center Hospital at Tel
Hashomer, Affiliated to the Sackler Faculty of
Medicine, Tel Aviv University, Ramat Gan, Israel

JAMES H. CALANDRUCCIO, MD
Assistant Professor, Department of
Orthopaedic Surgery and Biomedical
Engineering, University of
Tennessee–Campbell Clinic; Staff Physician,
Campbell Clinic, Inc, Memphis, Tennessee

CARA CIPRIANO, MD
Assistant Professor, Department of
Orthopedics, Washington University in
St Louis, St Louis, Missouri

KEITH P. CONNOLLY, MD
Resident, Department of Orthopaedic
Surgery, University of Pennsylvania,
Philadelphia, Pennsylvania

BRIAN CURTIN, MD
Assistant Professor, OrthoCarolina, Charlotte,
North Carolina

JAIME R. DENNING, MD
Assistant Professor, Orthopaedic Surgery,
Cincinnati Children's Hospital Medical Center,
Cincinnati, Ohio

NICHOLAS ERDLE, MD
Resident, Department of Orthopedics, Naval
Medical Center, Portsmouth, Maine

THOMAS K. FEHRING, MD
Surgeon, OrthoCarolina Hip & Knee Center,
Charlotte, North Carolina

HEATHER E. GOTHA, MD
Baylor University Medical Center, Dallas,
Texas

LANGDON A. HARTSOCK, MD
Department of Orthopaedics, Medical
University of South Carolina, Charleston,
South Carolina

ROBERT E. HOLMES, MD
Department of Orthopaedics, Medical
University of South Carolina, Charleston,
South Carolina

CHRISTOPHER M. HOPKINS, MD
Department of Orthopaedic Surgery and
Biomedical Engineering, University of
Tennessee–Campbell Clinic, Memphis,
Tennessee

KAI LI, MD
Resident, Department of Orthopedics,
Virginia Commonwealth University, Richmond,
Virginia

BENJAMIN M. MAUCK, MD
Hand and Upper Extremity Surgery, Campbell
Clinic; Clinical Instructor, Department of
Orthopedic Surgery, University of Tennessee
Health Science Center, Memphis, Tennessee

SAMIR MEHTA, MD
Chief of Orthopaedic Trauma; Associate
Professor, Department of Orthopaedic
Surgery, University of Pennsylvania,
Philadelphia, Pennsylvania

JEFFREY G. MOKRIS, MD
Surgeon, OrthoCarolina Hip & Knee Center,
Charlotte, North Carolina

SUSAN M. ODUM, PhD
Senior Research Scientist, OrthoCarolina
Research Institute, Charlotte, North Carolina

JOSHUA C. ROZELL, MD
Resident, Department of Orthopaedic
Surgery, University of Pennsylvania,
Philadelphia, Pennsylvania

NACHSHON SHAZAR, MD
Department of Orthopedic Surgery, Chaim
Sheba Medical Center Hospital at Tel
Hashomer, Affiliated to the Sackler Faculty of
Medicine, Tel Aviv University, Ramat Gan,
Israel

BRYAN D. SPRINGER, MD
Surgeon, OrthoCarolina Hip & Knee Center,
Charlotte, North Carolina

LOUIS S. STRYKER, MD
Assistant Professor, Joint Reconstruction,
Department of Orthopaedic Surgery and
Rehabilitation, University of Texas Health
Science Center San Antonio, San Antonio,
Texas

SHAY TENENBAUM, MD
Department of Orthopedic Surgery, Chaim
Sheba Medical Center Hospital at Tel
Hashomer, Affiliated to the Sackler Faculty of
Medicine, Tel Aviv University, Ramat Gan,
Israel

DAVID N. VEGARI, MD
Surgeon, Lankenau Medical Center,
Wynnewood, Pennsylvania

SCOTT YANG, MD
Assistant Professor of Orthopaedics
and Rehabilitation, Doernbecher
Children's Hospital, Oregon Health and
Science University, Portland,
Oregon

JACOB R. ZIDE, MD
Assistant Professor of Orthopaedics at UT
Southwestern and Texas A&M; Baylor
University Medical Center, Dallas,
Texas

CONTENTS

Adult Reconstruction
Patrick C. Toy

Total knee arthroplasty occasionally does not meet expectations. This randomized clinical trial assessed the effect of restoration of the native patellofemoral
height on clinical outcomes. Group I underwent standard patellar bone resection; group II underwent modified patellar bone resection that adjusted the
amount of anterior condylar bone removed and the anterior flange thickness.
There were no differences in anterior knee pain, Western Ontario and McMaster Universities Arthritis Index scores, or Knee Injury and Osteoarthritis
Outcome Score scores. Patellofemoral compartment height restoration versus
patellar height alone does not appear to significantly reduce pain or improve
function.

The optimal strategy for postoperative deep venous thrombosis prophylaxis
remains controversial in hip and knee arthroplasty. Warfarin causes transient
hypercoagulability; however, the optimal timing of treatment remains unclear.
We evaluated the effects of preoperative versus postoperative warfarin therapy with a primary endpoint of perioperative change in hemoglobin. Warfarin
was dosed according to a standard nomogram. No difference in perioperative
hemoglobin change was observed. The preoperative group demonstrated
higher INRs. Initiation of warfarin preoperatively was not associated with any
difference in perioperative hemoglobin change. Larger studies are needed
to determine whether the risk of adverse events is increased with either
strategy.

This article describes a study comparing 30-day readmission rates between patients undergoing outpatient versus inpatient total hip (THA) and knee (TKA)
arthroplasty. A retrospective review of 137 patients undergoing outpatient total
joint arthroplasty (TJA) and 106 patients undergoing inpatient (minimum 2-day
hospital stay) TJA was conducted. Unplanned hospital readmissions and unplanned episodes of care were recorded. All patients completed a telephone
survey. Seven inpatients and 16 outpatients required hospital readmission or an
unplanned episode of care following hospital discharge. Readmission rates
were higher for TKA than THA. The authors found no statistical differences in
30-day readmission or unplanned care episodes.

Trauma
John C. Weinlein

The optimal treatment of open fractures continues to be an area of debate in the orthopedic literature. Recent research has challenged the dictum that open fractures should be debrided within 6 hours of injury. However, the expedient administration of intravenous antibiotics remains of paramount importance in infection prevention. Multiple factors, including fracture severity, thoroughness of debridement, time to initial treatment, and antibiotic administration, among other variables, contribute to the incidence of infection and complicate identifying an optimal time to debridement.

Better understanding of the biology of heterotopic ossification (HO) formation will lead to treatment and prevention modalities that can be directed specifically at the cellular level. Early identification of HO precursor cells and target genes may provide prognostic value that guides individualized prophylactic treatment. Better understanding of molecular signaling and proteomics variability will allow surgeons to individualize preemptive treatment to suppress inflammation and formation of HO. Careful surgical technique to avoid muscle damage is important. Damaged muscle should be debrided as a prophylactic measure. Hemostasis and avoidance of a postoperative hematoma may decrease the chance of formation of HO.

Pediatrics
Jeffrey R. Sawyer

Midshaft clavicle fractures in adolescents are common. Recent literature in adults fractures favors open reduction and plate fixation for significantly displaced and/or shortened midshaft clavicle fractures, although whether this applies to adolescents remains debatable. This article reviews the current literature and controversy in the management of displaced adolescent clavicle fractures.

Ankle fractures account for 5% and foot fractures account for approximately 8% of fractures in children. Some complications are evident early in the treatment or natural history of foot and ankle fractures. Other complications do not become apparent until weeks, months, or years after the original fracture. The incidence of long-term sequelae like posttraumatic arthritis from childhood foot and ankle fractures is poorly studied because decades or lifelong follow-up has frequently not been accomplished. This article discusses a variety of complications associated with foot and ankle fractures in children or the treatment of these injuries.

Upper Extremity
Benjamin M. Mauck and James H. Calandruccio

> The olecranon process, coronoid process, and greater sigmoid notch are important components of the complex proximal ulna. Along with providing bony stability to the ulnohumeral joint, the proximal ulna serves as the attachment site of many important muscles and ligaments that impart soft tissue stability to the elbow joint. Management of proximal ulnar fractures continues to evolve as advances in imaging and anatomic and biomechanical studies have led to improvements in available implants; however, controversies remain, as shown in the current relevant literature.

Foot and Ankle
Benjamin J. Grear

> Posterior malleolus fractures vary in morphology. A computed tomography scan is imperative to evaluate fragment size, comminution, articular impaction, and syndesmotic disruption. Despite an increasing body of literature regarding posterior malleolus fractures, many questions remain unanswered. Although, historically, fragment size guided surgical fixation, it is becoming evident that fragment size should not solely dictate treatment. Surgical treatment should focus on restoring ankle joint structural integrity, which includes restoring articular congruity, correcting posterior talar translation, addressing articular impaction, removing osteochondral debris, and establishing syndesmotic stability.

> Displaced intraarticular fractures of the calcaneus represent a technically challenging injury. Although there is conflicting evidence regarding advantages and disadvantages of operative versus nonoperative treatment, a growing body of literature suggests operative management with near-anatomic reduction of the posterior facet and restoration of overall calcaneal morphology offers greater potential for superior short- and long-term outcomes. A thorough understanding of calcaneal anatomy, fracture pattern, and associated injuries, along with careful selection of surgical approach and timing to surgery are critical to minimize the risk of complication and maximize potential for optimal outcomes.

CONTROVERSIES IN FRACTURE CARE

THE CLINICS ARE AVAILABLE ONLINE!

Access your subscription at:
www.theclinics.com

PREFACE

Controversies in Fracture Care

Although fractures are the most frequently treated orthopedic injuries, and have been for centuries, some aspects of their care remain controversial and other areas become controversial as newer information comes to light. This issue of *Orthopedic Clinics of North America* highlights a few of these areas.

The first three articles, although they deal with total joint arthroplasty rather than fractures, highlight the importance of patellofemoral offset in total knee arthroplasty, controversies in deep vein thrombosis prophylaxis with warfarin, and inpatient compared with outpatient arthroplasty.

In the next section, Rozell, Connolly, and Mehta challenge the long-standing dictum that open fractures should be debrided within 6 hours of injury by describing a myriad of other factors that affect the frequency of infection and complicate identification of an optimal time to debridement.

One area in which new knowledge may change treatment methods is that of posttraumatic heterotopic ossification (HO). Historically, radiation therapy and medications such as indomethacin have been used for prophylaxis, but Barfield, Holmes, and Hartsock provide information about the biology of HO and suggest that a better understanding of molecular signaling and proteomics variability may lead to individualized prophylactic protocols to suppress the formation of HO.

Although most fractures in children and adolescents heal without difficulty, midshaft clavicular fractures in adolescents have come under scrutiny because of less than optimal results with nonoperative treatment. Yang and Andras review the current controversy in the management of these fractures. Foot and ankle fractures are other entities that may seem benign in children but can have long-term adverse effects. Denning discusses a variety of complications associated with these fractures in children. Hopkins, Calandruccio, and Mauck then discuss controversies in fractures of the proximal ulna. Tenenbaum, Shazar, Bruck, and Bariteau, and Gotha and Zide discuss the treatment of posterior malleolar and calcaneal fractures in adults.

Overall, this issue provides much up-to-date information and highlights a number of controversies in the treatment of fractures. The authors and I hope this information will be beneficial to our readers as they determine the optimal care for their patients.

Frederick M. Azar, MD
Professor, Department of Orthopaedic Surgery
and Biomedical Engineering
University of Tennessee–Campbell Clinic
1211 Union Avenue, Suite 510
Memphis, TN 38104, USA
E-mail address:
fazar@campbellclinic.com

http://dx.doi.org/10.1016/j.ocl.2016.10.001
0030-5898/17/© 2016 Published by Elsevier Inc.

Adult Reconstruction

Role of Patellofemoral Offset in Total Knee Arthroplasty: A Randomized Trial

Louis S. Stryker, MD[a], Susan M. Odum, PhD[b],
Bryan D. Springer, MD[c],*, Thomas K. Fehring, MD[c]

KEYWORDS

- Total knee arthroplasty • Patellofemoral joint • Subject outcome assessment
- Treatment outcome • Randomized controlled trial

KEY POINTS

- The current study sought to establish if restoration of the overall patellofemoral joint thickness resulted in improved pain scores and function following primary total knee arthroplasty (TKA).
- There were no differences between groups in anterior knee pain, Western Ontario and McMaster Universities Arthritis Index (WOMAC) scores, or Knee Injury and Osteoarthritis Outcome Score (KOOS) scores.
- Overall, patellofemoral compartment height restoration versus patellar height alone does not seem to significantly reduce pain or improve function following TKA.

INTRODUCTION

Patient satisfaction following total knee arthroplasty (TKA) is inconsistent and frequently does not meet the expectations of patients, with as few as 4% of patients rating themselves as "very happy" with their outcome, despite excellent survivorship.[1] Therefore, understanding the causes for this lack of satisfaction and improving patient-perceived outcomes is critical, not only to better meet patient expectations but also with the understanding that these patient-reported outcomes will be published and potentially tied to reimbursement in the near future.

Anterior knee pain is a major contributor to patient dissatisfaction following TKA and remains a largely unsolved problem. In a study by Meftah and colleagues,[2] one-third of all TKA subjects experienced mild-to-moderate anterior knee pain at 1-year follow-up. This pain persisted in 30% of previously symptomatic subjects at 10 years, with 10% of previously asymptomatic subjects developing new onset anterior knee pain. Multiple technique and implant-related causes have been previously described, including instability, component rotation, component characteristics, and overstuffing of the patellofemoral joint.[3–10] Anatomic considerations have also been examined. Kohl and colleagues[11] found no correlation between patellar blood flow and anterior knee pain following TKA. Additionally, attempts to curb anterior knee pain through circumpatellar electrocautery denervation have had variable results.[12,13] Despite improvements in surgical

Disclosure Statement: One or more of the authors has received funding from DePuy (T.K. Fehring, B.D. Springer) and Stryker (B.D. Springer). The institution of the authors has received funding from Biomet, Corin, DePuy, Smith and Nephew, Stryker, and Zimmer.
[a] Joint Reconstruction, Department of Orthopaedic Surgery and Rehabilitation, University of Texas Health Science Center San Antonio, 7703 Floyd Curl Drive, MSC-7774, San Antonio, TX 78229, USA; [b] OrthoCarolina Research Institute, 2001 Vail Avenue, Suite 300, Charlotte, NC 28207, USA; [c] OrthoCarolina Hip & Knee Center, 2001 Vail Avenue, Suite 200A, Charlotte, NC 28207, USA
* Corresponding author.
E-mail address: Bryan.Springer@orthocarolina.com

techniques and advances in implant characteristics to more patellofemoral joint-friendly designs, anterior knee pain following TKA persists and largely remains an enigma.[14,15]

The patellofemoral joint is composed of the patella and the corresponding anterior aspect of the distal femur with which it articulates. During TKA, the anterior aspect of the distal femur is resected flush with the anterior femoral cortex and resurfaced with the anterior flange of the femoral component. In instances of patellar resurfacing, the patella is resected and an implant placed on its cut surface. Current surgical techniques call for restoration of the patellar thickness by removing a depth of patellar bone that corresponds with patellar implant thickness. This technique, however, does not account for the amount of anterior distal femoral bone that is resected and replaced by the femoral component. As a result, an emphasis is placed on restoring patellar thickness but not necessarily restoring the overall thickness of the native patellofemoral joint. Because a wide variation in anterior condyle anatomy has been previously described, there is a high likelihood that the native patellofemoral joint height is not reestablished during conventional TKA, either by overstuffing the patellofemoral joint or inadequately restoring the patellofemoral height.[16] Such inaccuracy may adversely affect knee function by altering the native extensor mechanism and its moment arm, either by creating laxity in the case of overresection or by over tightening the extensor mechanism if underresected.[17,18]

Because there is currently a lack of literature examining this issue, the authors pose the following research questions:

1. Does restoration of native overall patellofemoral height reduce pain following primary TKA?
2. Does restoration of native overall patellofemoral height improve function following primary TKA?

SUBJECTS AND METHODS
Subject Selection
Following institutional review board approval, a cohort of consecutive subjects undergoing elective primary TKA was prospectively randomized to either the experimental or control group. All patients presenting for primary TKA who had failed conservative management were included as study candidates. Patients were excluded if they were deemed candidates for unicompartmental knee arthroplasty, were undergoing

revision TKA, had preoperative angular deformities of greater than 15°, had patellar subluxation or dislocation on history or clinical or radiographic examination, or had severe patellar bone loss as determined by the operating surgeon. Clinical coordinators collected study data during preoperative and postoperative clinic visits. A random-number generator was used to randomize subjects to either the control group or experimental group in a 1 to 1 fashion. Subjects and clinical coordinators were blinded as to the group assignment. The performing statistician was also blinded to the groups.

Assuming an estimated anterior knee pain visual analog score (VAS) score of 15 in the control group and a VAS pain score of 5 in the experimental group, a 1-sided t-test assuming equal variance (standard deviation of 10 points) with an effect size Cohen's d of 1.0, and an alpha level of 0.05, an estimated 23 subjects were needed in each group for 90% power. Allowing for a 15% lost to follow-up rate, 26 subjects were enrolled into each group for a total of 52 subjects.

Forty-six subjects completed the study with at least 1 year of follow-up and were included in the analysis. Six subjects initially enrolled were excluded from analysis, including 2 subjects in group I and 1 subject in group II who did not return for their 1-year evaluation. An additional 2 subjects in group I were excluded from analysis because the patella was deemed to be too thin by the operating surgeon at the time of surgery to safely perform the patellar resection as required by the study. One subject in group II was excluded due to failure from infection before 1-year follow-up.

The final dataset consists of 22 subjects in group I, which includes of 15 women and 7 men. Group II was composed of 24 subjects, with 20 women and 4 men. The mean age of group I was 67 years (range, 50–78 years) with a mean age of 69 years in group II (range, 54–82 years). There were no statistical differences between groups in the demographic characteristics of the study subjects. The demographic data for each group are reported in Table 1.

Subjects in both groups underwent cemented, posterior stabilized, TKA performed through a standard medial parapatellar arthrotomy using gap-balancing technique by 1 of 2 fellowship-trained arthroplasty surgeons (Springer BD, Fehring TK). All patellae were resurfaced and a tourniquet was used in every case, inflated before incision, and released after curing of all cement. Primary total knee components from 2 different manufacturers (DePuy, Warsaw, IN, USA; and,

Table 1 Subject demographics					
	Number of Subjects	Mean Age (Range)	P-Value	Women/Men	P-Value
Group I	22	67 y (50–78)	.42	15/7	.22
Group II	24	69 y (54–82)	—	20/4	—

Stryker, Mahwah, NJ, USA) were used at the discretion of the operating surgeon.

In the control group (group I), the goal was to restore native patellar thickness. As such, the patella was measured by caliper and resected to a level such that the overall patellar thickness was restored following placement of the patellar component (Fig. 1). In the experimental group (group II), the goal was to restore the overall thickness of the native patellofemoral joint. To that end, the thickness of anterior distal femoral bone resected during standard distal femoral preparation was measured and subtracted from the thickness of the corresponding anterior aspect thickness of the femoral component (Fig. 2). The thickness of the native patella was then measured and the amount of patellar bone resected adjusted, such that the overall native patellofemoral joint thickness would be restored when accounting for the thickness of the patellar component and any differences between the amount of anterior distal femur and the corresponding anterior femoral component thickness. For example, if the amount of bone resected from the anterior condyle measured 10 mm and the thickness of the anterior flange of the component was 8 mm, 2 mm less bone was taken off the patella to recreate the overall thickness of the patellofemoral joint.

The mean intraoperative patellar height before resection was 23.48 mm (SD = 1.98 mm) in group I and 22.82 mm (SD = 2.03 mm) in group II ($P = .25$). The mean overall patellofemoral joint height, defined as the amount of anterior distal femoral bone resected plus the native patellar height, was 29.38 mm (SD = 3.38 mm) in group I and 29.58 mm (SD = 3.06 mm) in group II ($P = .83$). The mean patellar height following resection was 14.11 mm (SD = 1.35 mm) in group I and 13.7 mm (SD = 1.74 mm) in group II ($P = .36$). The mean change in patellar height following resection and component placement was +0.59 mm (SD = 0.56) in group I and +1.28 mm (SD = 1.1 mm) in group II ($P = .0075$). The change in overall patellofemoral height following placement of final components was +2.52 mm (SD = 1.96) in group I and +0.86 mm (SD = 1.06) in group II ($P = .005$) (Table 2).

Clinical Outcome Measures

Subjects were followed for 1 year postoperatively with the anterior knee pain VAS. Study subjects also completed the Knee Injury and Osteoarthritis Outcome Score (KOOS). Western Ontario and McMaster Universities Arthritis Index (WOMAC) total score as well as the WOMAC subscores were derived from the KOOS (Table 3).

Statistical Analysis

Statistical analyses were all performed using SAS software, version 9.2 (Cary, NC, USA). Univariate, descriptive statistics were calculated and included frequency, proportions, means, and standard deviations. Bivariate analyses were performed using a student t-test and chi-square test. A student t-test was used to determine differences in mean values between groups for the

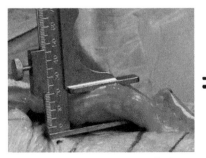 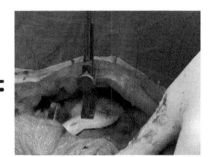

Fig. 1. Group I subjects had native patellar thickness restored by removing an amount of bone equal to the thickness of the patellar component.

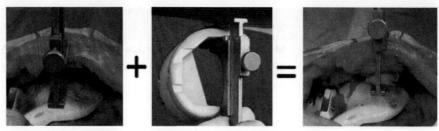

Fig. 2. Group II subjects had native patellofemoral compartment thickness restored. The amount of patellar bone resected was altered to account for the thickness of anterior distal femur resected.

following variables: subject age, patellar height, patellofemoral height, anterior knee pain VAS, KOOS subscores, and WOMAC subscores. A chi-square test was used to determine the difference in the proportions between men and women. An a priori 0.05 level of significance was used for all statistical tests.

RESULTS

The preoperative mean VAS pain score in group I was 49.52 versus 54.96 in group II (P = .55). Postoperative VAS pain scores decreased to 11.84 and 4.08 in groups I and II, respectively (P = .14). The preoperative WOMAC pain scores for groups I and II were 47.05 and 50.00 (P = .59), respectively; whereas postoperative WOMAC pain scores were 92.27 and 93.95 for groups I and II, respectively (P = .55). KOOS

pain scores for groups I and II were 43.18 and 47.22 (P = .47) preoperatively, improving to 91.41 and 91.08, respectively (P = .91).

In regard to knee function, the WOMAC total was 44.82 in group I and in group II it was 46.59 (P = .72) preoperatively, whereas postoperative scores were 89.26 for group I and 90.59 for group II (P = .65). For WOMAC stiffness, the preoperative value was 44.32 in group I and 36.97 in group II (P = .23), which improved postoperatively to 80.11 in group I and 79.16 in group II (P = .86). A WOMAC functions score of 42.58 was found in group I and 48.16 in group II, preoperatively. Postoperatively, these values changed in group I to 91.04 and group II to 93.26 (P = .39). Function daily living (DL) in group I was 42.58 preoperatively, whereas in group II it was 48.16 (P = .35), which changed to 91.04 in group I and 93.26 in group II

Table 2
Differences between native patellar thickness, native patellofemoral height, postresection patellar thickness, change in patellar height after resurfacing, and change in patellofemoral height

	Mean (mm)	Standard Deviation (mm)	P-Value
Native Patellar Thickness			
Group 1	23.48	1.9816	.25
Group 2	22.82	2.0304	—
Overall Patellofemoral Height			
Group 1	29.38	3.38	.83
Group 2	29.58	3.06	—
Posresection Patellar Thickness			
Group 1	14.11	1.35	.36
Group 2	13.7	1.74	—
Change in Patellar Height After Resurfacing			
Group 1	0.59	0.56	.0075
Group 2	1.28	1.1	—
Change in Patellofemoral Height			
Group 1	2.518	1.96	.0005
Group 2	0.86	1.06	—

Table 3
Pain and function scores preoperatively and at annual follow-up for groups I and II

| | Preoperative | | Annual | |
	Mean	P-Value	Mean	P-Value
VAS Pain				
Group 1	49.52	.55	11.84	.14
Group 2	54.96	—	4.08	—
WOMAC Total				
Group 1	44.82	.72	89.26	.65
Group 2	46.59	—	90.59	—
WOMAC Pain				
Group 1	47.05	.59	92.27	.55
Group 2	50.00	—	93.95	—
WOMAC Stiff				
Group 1	44.32	.23	80.11	.86
Group 2	36.97	—	79.16	—
WOMAC Functions				
Group 1	42.58	.35	91.04	.39
Group 2	48.16	—	93.26	—
Function DL				
Group 1	42.58	.35	91.04	.39
Group 2	48.16	—	93.26	—
Function SRA				
Group 1	10.00	.68	62.50	.25
Group 2	11.87	—	73.54	—
KOOS Symptoms				
Group 1	49.68	.21	88.47	.43
Group 2	41.67	—	85.86	—
KOOS Pain				
Group 1	43.18	.47	91.41	.91
Group 2	47.22	—	91.08	—
KOOS Quality of Life				
Group 1	22.44	.88	82.67	.41
Group 2	23.18	—	77.86	—

(P = .39). Function sport and recreation activity (SRA) preoperatively was 10.00 in group I and 11.87 in group II (P = .68). Postoperative function SRA improved in group I to 62.50 and in group II to 73.54 (P = .25). Preoperative KOOS symptoms for group I was 49.68 and for group II 41.67 (P = .21) and postoperatively was 88.47 in group I and 85.86 in group II (P = .43). KOOS quality of life (QOL) for group I was 22.44 and 23.18 for group II (P = .88) preoperatively. Postoperative KOOS QOL scores were 82.67 for group I and 77.86 for group II (P = .41).

SUMMARY

Most previous investigations regarding the patellofemoral joint in TKA involved femoral component design and rotation, as well as whether or not the patella was resurfaced, particularly in terms of anterior knee pain and patellar thickness.[3–5,10,14,19–23] The clinical significance of overstuffing or understuffing the patellofemoral compartment, however, remains debatable.[19,22,24–27] The current study sought to establish if restoration of the overall patellofemoral joint thickness, as opposed to the native patellar thickness, resulted in improved pain scores and function following primary TKA.

The authors recognize the current study's limitations. First, the potential for type II beta error exists and, potentially, a larger study size might identify a statistically significant difference between the 2 groups. In addition, the patients who may benefit most from this technique are those who have comparatively large anterior condyles (large males with large anterior posterior dimension of the femur) resected during TKA and, therefore, the overall patellofemoral height is not adequately restored using conventional patellar preparation. Given the current study design, we are not able to address this question. Also, this study was designed to assess for differences in anterior knee pain and function. An analysis of quadriceps function and efficiency, however, may reveal more subtle differences between the 2 groups. Furthermore, the patellofemoral compartment encountered at the time of TKA may not accurately reflect the true overall patellofemoral height in a nondiseased state. This may have affected the results, despite exclusion of subjects with significant patellar bone loss, and because native patellar height and overall patellofemoral joint thickness was successfully restored to within 1 mm in group I and group II, respectively. The height of the patellofemoral compartment directly anterior to the distal femur also may not be the most appropriate area for evaluation. Instead, the thickness of the patellofemoral compartment as it engages the trochlear groove in early flexion may be more important as a contributor to anterior knee pain due to contact stresses.[8,27,28] Furthermore, the current study describes restoration of the patellofemoral joint, a static measurement, and may not accurately reflect what happens kinematically in vivo.[29–31] The current study also does not account for any change in the joint line or patellar tendon length, which may also affect outcomes.[32] Finally, design differences that can affect the extensor moment arm and, therefore, alter patellofemoral contact forces, were not controlled for in the study design.[17]

Pierson and colleagues,[26] in a large retrospective study, examined a multitude of factors involved in overstuffing the patellofemoral joint and their association with outcomes. The investigators discovered that increases in anterior femoral offset resulted in no significant change in Knee Society pain score.[26] The study did not report, however, on changes in outcomes related to changes in patellar thickness and anterior femoral offset (patellofemoral joint thickness). Similarly, the current study did not identify statistically significant differences in pain between the experimental and control groups. There was, however, a trend toward significance noted in the anterior knee VAS pain score.

A limited number of studies have examined the functional role of the patellofemoral joint thickness in TKA. Mihalko and colleagues,[33] in a cadaveric study, examined the role of increasing anterior femoral component thickness on range of motion. The investigators found that increased anterior buildups resulted in reduced range of motion; however, the clinical significance of this finding was unclear.[33] In the same study reporting on Knee Society pain scores, Pierson and colleagues[26] reported a small negative effect on knee function along with an increased likelihood for lateral retinacular release. The current study was unable to establish any improvement in function in any of the outcome measures used when the overall patellofemoral height was restored as opposed to the native patellar height.

Similar to previously reported results, restoration of overall patellofemoral joint thickness, as opposed to restoration of native patellar height, does not seem to significantly affect outcomes of primary TKA, although there was a trend toward improved anterior knee pain.

ACKNOWLEDGMENTS

The authors thank all of the staff of the OrthoCarolina Research Institute. Specifically, the authors would like to thank Ben Connell for his dedication as the study coordinator.

REFERENCES

1. Beverland D. Patient satisfaction following TKA: bless them all! Orthopedics 2010;33(9):657.
2. Meftah M, Ranawat AS, Ranawat CS. The natural history of anterior knee pain in 2 posterior-stabilized, modular total knee arthroplasty designs. J Arthroplasty 2011;26(8):1145–8.
3. Barrack RL, Schrader T, Bertot AJ, et al. Component rotation and anterior knee pain after total knee arthroplasty. Clin Orthop Relat Res 2001;392:46–55.
4. Berger RA, Crossett LS, Jacobs JJ, et al. Malrotation causing patellofemoral complications after total knee arthroplasty. Clin Orthop Relat Res 1998; 356:144–53.

5. Frye BM, Floyd MW, Pham DC, et al. Effect of femoral component design on patellofemoral crepitance and patella clunk syndrome after posterior-stabilized total knee arthroplasty. J Arthroplasty 2012;27(6):1166–70.

6. Hozack WJ, Rothman RH, Booth RE Jr, et al. The patellar clunk syndrome. A complication of posterior stabilized total knee arthroplasty. Clin Orthop Relat Res 1989;241:203–8.

7. Pagnano MW, Hanssen AD, Lewallen DG, et al. Flexion instability after primary posterior cruciate retaining total knee arthroplasty. Clin Orthop Relat Res 1998;356:39–46.

8. Rand JA. The patellofemoral joint in total knee arthroplasty. J Bone Joint Surg Am 1994;76(4):612–20.

9. Rand JA. Extensor mechanism complications following total knee arthroplasty. J Bone Joint Surg Am 2004;86(9):2062–72.

10. Scuderi GR, Insall JN, Scott NW. Patellofemoral pain after total knee arthroplasty. J Am Acad Orthop Surg 1994;2(5):239–46.

11. Kohl S, Evangelopoulos DS, Hartel M, et al. Anterior knee pain after total knee arthroplasty: does it correlate with patellar blood flow? Knee Surg Sports Traumatol Arthrosc 2011;19(9):1453–9.

12. Baliga S, McNair CJ, Barnett KJ, et al. Does circumpatellar electrocautery improve the outcome after total knee replacement?: a prospective, randomised, blinded controlled trial. J Bone Joint Surg Br 2012;94(9):1228–33.

13. van Jonbergen HP, Scholtes VA, van Kampen A, et al. A randomised, controlled trial of circumpatellar electrocautery in total knee replacement without patellar resurfacing. J Bone Joint Surg Br 2011;93(8):1054–9.

14. Indelli PF, Marcucci M, Cariello D, et al. Contemporary femoral designs in total knee arthroplasty: effects on the patello-femoral congruence. Int Orthop 2012;36(6):1167–73.

15. Mahoney OM, McClung CD, dela Rosa MA, et al. The effect of total knee arthroplasty design on extensor mechanism function. J Arthroplasty 2002;17(4):416–21.

16. Fehring TK, Odum SM, Hughes J, et al. Differences between the sexes in the anatomy of the anterior condyle of the knee. J Bone Joint Surg Am 2009;91(10):2335–41.

17. Browne C, Hermida JC, Bergula A, et al. Patellofemoral forces after total knee arthroplasty: effect of extensor moment arm. Knee 2005;12(2):81–8.

18. D'Lima DD, Poole C, Chadha H, et al. Quadriceps moment arm and quadriceps forces after total knee arthroplasty. Clin Orthop Relat Res 2001;392:213–20.

19. Bengs BC, Scott RD. The effect of patellar thickness on intraoperative knee flexion and patellar tracking in total knee arthroplasty. J Arthroplasty 2006;21(5):650–5.

20. Fitzpatrick CK, Kim RH, Ali AA, et al. Effects of resection thickness on mechanics of resurfaced patellae. J Biomech 2013;46(9):1568–75.

21. Hsu HC, Luo ZP, Rand JA, et al. Influence of patellar thickness on patellar tracking and patellofemoral contact characteristics after total knee arthroplasty. J Arthroplasty 1996;11(1):69–80.

22. Koh JS, Yeo SJ, Lee BP, et al. Influence of patellar thickness on results of total knee arthroplasty: does a residual bony patellar thickness of <or=12 mm lead to poorer clinical outcome and increased complication rates? J Arthroplasty 2002;17(1):56–61.

23. Steinbruck A, Schroder C, Woiczinski M, et al. Patellofemoral contact patterns before and after total knee arthroplasty: an in vitro measurement. Biomed Eng Online 2013;12:58.

24. Ghosh KM, Merican AM, Iranpour F, et al. The effect of overstuffing the patellofemoral joint on the extensor retinaculum of the knee. Knee Surg Sports Traumatol Arthrosc 2009;17(10):1211–6.

25. Mofidi A, Bajada S, Holt MD, et al. Functional relevance of patellofemoral thickness before and after unicompartmental patellofemoral replacement. Knee 2012;19(3):180–4.

26. Pierson JL, Ritter MA, Keating EM, et al. The effect of stuffing the patellofemoral compartment on the outcome of total knee arthroplasty. J Bone Joint Surg Am 2007;89(10):2195–203.

27. Stiehl JB, Komistek RD, Dennis DA, et al. Kinematics of the patellofemoral joint in total knee arthroplasty. J Arthroplasty 2001;16(6):706–14.

28. Ahmed AM, Burke DL, Yu A. In-vitro measurement of static pressure distribution in synovial joints–Part II: Retropatellar surface. J Biomech Eng 1983;105(3):226–36.

29. Ahmed AM, Burke DL, Hyder A. Force analysis of the patellar mechanism. J Orthop Res 1987;5(1):69–85.

30. Baldini A, Anderson JA, Cerulli-Mariani P, et al. Patellofemoral evaluation after total knee arthroplasty. Validation of a new weight-bearing axial radiographic view. J Bone Joint Surg Am 2007;89(8):1810–7.

31. Draper CE, Besier TF, Fredericson M, et al. Differences in patellofemoral kinematics between weight-bearing and non-weight-bearing conditions in patients with patellofemoral pain. J Orthop Res 2011;29(3):312–7.

32. Junior LH, Soares LF, Goncalves MB, et al. Relationship between patellar height and range of motion after total knee arthroplasty. Rev Bras Ortop 2011;46(4):408–11.

33. Mihalko W, Fishkin Z, Krackow K. Patellofemoral overstuff and its relationship to flexion after total knee arthroplasty. Clin Orthop Relat Res 2006;449:283–7.

Preoperative Versus Postoperative Initiation of Warfarin Therapy in Patients Undergoing Total Hip and Knee Arthroplasty

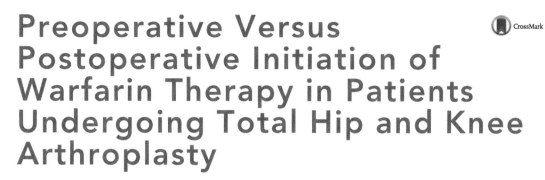 CrossMark

Cara Cipriano, MD[a], Nicholas Erdle, MD[b], Kai Li, MD[c], Brian Curtin, MD[d],*

KEYWORDS

• Warfarin • Dosing regimen • Anticoagulation • Perioperative blood loss

KEY POINTS

• Initiation of warfarin therapy on the night before surgery versus the night after surgery was associated with significantly decreased drain output and earlier increases in postoperative International Normalized Ratio (INR).
• We did not observe a difference in perioperative change in hemoglobin.
• We were unable to detect any difference in complication rates between groups.

INTRODUCTION

The optimal strategy for postoperative deep venous thrombosis (DVT) prophylaxis remains a controversial topic in hip and knee arthroplasty. Although it has been widely accepted that some form is required, a consensus on the ideal modality has not been established.[1] The benefits of chemical DVT prophylaxis must be balanced against the risks of anticoagulation in the early postoperative period, because increased bleeding can necessitate transfusions as well as lead to hematomas and other wound healing complications.

Warfarin therapy is the most commonly used form of chemical DVT prophylaxis after hip and knee arthroplasty in the United States.[2] It is usually administered beginning the evening after surgery and titrated according to International Normalized Ratio (INR) with a target range of 1.6 to 3.0, depending on the institution and surgeon.[2] It acts by preventing the carboxylation of vitamin K–dependent clotting factors in the liver; however, it first affects anticoagulant protein C and S, leading to an interval of transient hypercoagulability. Although the risk of DVT formation may begin at the time of surgery or during the early postoperative period, patients are unprotected until their INRs reach appropriate levels[3]; thus, the optimal timing of warfarin treatment with respect to surgery remains unclear.

We evaluated the effects of preoperative versus postoperative initiation of warfarin therapy on postoperative INR, perioperative blood loss, and related complications.

PATIENTS AND METHODS

This quasirandomized controlled study included all primary, elective total hip and knee

All work was related to this study was performed at Virginia Commonwealth University, Richmond, VA.
No conflicts of interest to report for any author involved in this study.
[a] Department of Orthopedics, Washington University in St Louis, St Louis, MO, USA; [b] Department of Orthopedics, Naval Medical Center, Portsmouth, ME, USA; [c] Department of Orthopedics, Virginia Commonwealth University, Richmond, VA, USA; [d] OrthoCarolina, 2001 Vail Avenue, Suite 200A, Charlotte, NC 28207, USA
* Corresponding author.
E-mail address: bmcurt01@gmail.com

arthroplasties (THA, TKA) performed by the senior author (BC) at a single institution over a 12-month period (January 2012–January 2013). Patients were assigned to begin taking warfarin the night before surgery or the night after surgery based on day of the week evaluated in clinic; those seen on Mondays and Wednesdays were prescribed 5 mg warfarin the evening before surgery, whereas those seen on Friday began warfarin on the evening after surgery. An a priori power analysis was performed to ensure appropriate sample size to detect a difference of 0.5 g/dL in perioperative change in hemoglobin between groups, given an alpha level of 0.05 and beta of 0.80. The results indicated that 64 patients would be required in each group, or at least 140 total when allowing for an estimated 10% exclusion rate.

The demographic distribution of patients assigned to each group is shown in Table 1. Preoperative hemoglobin levels were measured on all patients within 2 weeks of surgery. Morphine spinal anesthesia was routinely used, and all TKAs were performed using a tourniquet, which was inflated at the time of incision and deflated before closure. A single medium HemoVac drain (10 French/0.125 in/0.32 cm diameter) was placed at the end of each case and discontinued on the morning of postoperative day (POD) 1. All patients received 5 mg of warfarin at 10 PM on the evening after surgery (6–12 hours postoperatively), and a standard nomogram was used to titrate warfarin dosing according to INR levels in both patient groups thereafter. The surgeon and other staff were blinded to the patient's anticoagulation protocols at the time of surgery and throughout their hospitalizations.

After receiving appropriate Institutional Review Board approval, the electronic medical records for patients in the study population were retrospectively reviewed for INR levels (on POD 1 and 2), drain outputs (on POD 1, when all drains were removed), and change between preoperative and postoperative hemoglobin levels (on PODs 1 and 2). Patients were monitored clinically, but no Doppler studies or other screening modalities were performed to detect asymptomatic DVTs. The number of adverse events related to anticoagulation (wound healing complications, hematomas [abnormal swelling and fluid accumulation within the knee], epidural complications, and transfusions) or thrombosis (symptomatic DVT, pulmonary embolus) was also noted. These outcomes were compared between patient populations using a χ^2 test for categorical variables (wound healing complications, hematomas, and transfusions) and the Student t test for continuous variables (postoperative INR, drain output, and change between preoperative and postoperative hemoglobin levels). Adverse events (transfusions, hematomas, epidural complications, symptomatic DVT, and pulmonary embolus) were compared using the 2-tailed Fischer's exact test.

RESULTS

Of the 177 patients initially reviewed, 12 were excluded: 7 receiving chronic anticoagulation for treatment of another condition, 3 undergoing simultaneous procedures that would likely increase blood loss (2 significant hardware removals and 1 contralateral core decompression), and 2 with medical contraindications to warfarin (1 hemophiliac, 1 intolerance). Of the remaining 165 cases (108 THA, 57 TKA) available for study, 73 were prescribed warfarin preoperatively (49 THA, 24 TKA) and 92 postoperatively (59 THA, 33 TKA). Patients were evenly distributed between groups in terms of gender and hip versus knee arthroplasty ($P = .3429$ and $P = .7431$, respectively), although those who received postoperative warfarin were slightly older (mean 59.6 compared with 54.4 years; $P = .0034$; see Table 1). Five patients from the study group and 2 patients from the control group were discharged on POD 1 and therefore excluded from the analysis of INR and hemoglobin on POD 2. In addition, drain outputs were not reliably documented in 9 patients from the preoperative treatment group (6 not recorded, 3 fell out) and 6 patients from the postoperative treatment group (5 not recorded, 1 fell out), so these patients were excluded from the analysis of drain output.

No difference in perioperative change in hemoglobin was observed between groups on either POD 1 (mean, 3.279 vs 3.377; $P = .6824$) or POD 2 (mean, 4.0 vs 4.12; $P = .6831$). The study

Table 1
Demographic distribution of patients assigned to preoperative compared with postoperative initiation of warfarin treatment

	Study Group	Control Group	P
Total hip arthroplasty (n)	49	59	.7431
Total knee arthroplasty (n)	24	33	
Male (n)	29	45	.3429
Female (n)	43	47	
Age (y), mean	59.6	54.4	.0034

group demonstrated higher INRs on POD 1 (mean, 1.18 vs 1.12; P = .0023) and POD 2 (mean, 1.46 vs 1.31; P = .0006), with more patients achieving therapeutic INR ($\geq$1.8) by POD 2 (7.9% compared with 3.4%). This group was also found to have statistically significantly lower drain outputs (mean, 185.4 vs 268.7; P = .0025). Nine transfusions (4 study patients, 5 control patients), 3 hematomas (1 study patient, 2 control patients), 1 pulmonary embolus (study patient), 0 other symptomatic DVTs, and 0 epidural-related complications occurred; no difference in the rate of these events could be detected given the numbers available for study (Table 2).

DISCUSSION

The critical importance of DVT prophylaxis after THA and TKA has been well-established; however, the optimal agent and time of initiation to minimize both thrombotic and bleeding events remain widely debated. The ideal form of prophylaxis would provide anticoagulation during the period of greatest risk for thrombosis without increasing rates of wound healing complications, hematomas, and acute blood loss anemia necessitating transfusion.

Although thrombi theoretically begin to form intraoperatively with the combination of venous stasis and surgical trauma, the majority seem to develop in the early postoperative period and may continue to evolve over the ensuing weeks or months,[4,5] potentially leading to readmission or delayed complications.[6,7] To address this concern, the optimal timing of therapy using low-molecular-weight heparin and other relatively new anticoagulants for THA and TKA has been researched extensively.[3,8–14] The aggregate of this literature indicates that preoperative initiation is not necessary for effective prophylaxis, that initiation between 2 hours preoperative and 6 hours postoperatively increases the risk of major bleeds, and that initiation at 6 hours postoperatively is both safe and likely more efficacious than delayed administration at 12 to 24 hours.[11,12] These findings suggest that anticoagulation is less beneficial, or even potentially harmful, during and immediately after surgery itself, but extended delays may be less effective in preventing the development of thrombus.

The issue of anticoagulation timing has not been addressed with respect to warfarin, although it is the most common form of DVT prophylaxis used by members of the American Association of Hip and Knee Surgeons.[2] Warfarin therapy is typically initiated on the night after surgery; however, its mechanism of action is known to cause transient hypercoagulability owing to suppression of proteins C and S that precedes suppression of vitamin K–dependent clotting factors.[15,16] According to the literature as described, this initial hypercoagulability may be more advantageous during the period of greatest blood loss (ie, intraoperatively and immediately postoperatively) than during the days after surgery, when the patient might be at risk for thrombus development and propagation.

Our study did not identify an advantage for one warfarin-dosing strategy over the other, although a significant decrease in drain output was observed in the group that received preoperative warfarin (P = .0025). Mean output for the preoperative treatment group was 185.4 mL compared with 268.7 mL for the postoperative treatment group, resulting in an average difference of 83.3 mL that we consider clinically relevant. We also observed statistically significantly higher INRs in the study population on both POD 1 and 2 (P = .0023 and P = .0006, respectively); although the difference may not be clinically significant at that time point, it does suggest that the study group would reach therapeutic INR levels for DVT prophylaxis 1 day

Table 2
Effects of preoperative compared with postoperative initiation of warfarin therapy on patient INR, drain output, and perioperative drop in hemoglobin, as well as pertinent complication rates

	Study Group	Control Group	P
INR (mean, POD 1)	1.18	1.12	.0023
INR (mean, POD 2)	1.46	1.31	.0006
Drain output (mean)	185.4	268.7	.0025
Change in hemoglobin (mean, POD 1)	3.28	3.38	.6824
Change in hemoglobin (mean, POD 2)	4.00	4.12	.6831
Transfusions (n)	4	5	1.000
Hematomas (n)	1	2	1.000
Pulmonary emboli (n)	1	0	.4398
Symptomatic DVT (n)	0	0	n/a
Epidural complications (n)	0	0	n/a

Abbreviations: DVT, deep vein thrombosis; INR, International Normalized Ratio; POD, postoperative day.

sooner, as expected. Given the numbers available for study, no difference in the rates of thrombotic or bleeding complications could be detected.

This study has several limitations that must be acknowledged. Patients were not randomized strictly, but assigned to their treatment groups based on clinic day of the week in a quasiexperimental observational study design. Mean age was slightly younger in the study group (54.4 vs 59.6 years; $P = .0034$); however, this difference would not likely impact our results, and the patient distribution was otherwise even with respect to gender and hip versus knee arthroplasty ($P = .3429$ and $P = .7431$, respectively). Nine patients (12.3%) in the study group and 6 (6.5%) in the control group were excluded from analysis of drain output, primarily owing to insufficient documentation, and these data were considered missing completely at random. Most important, perhaps, a larger sample population would be needed to compare these warfarin dosing strategies in terms of rare but important complications related to bleeding or thrombosis.

In addition to these study-specific limitations, the evaluation of perioperative bleeding is subject to several inherent challenges. Minor discrepancies in surgical technique, patient size, or difficulty of the case can contribute to rates of intraoperative or postoperative blood loss. Serum hemoglobin may be affected by the hydration status of the patient, which in turn depends on several variables, such as the volume of intravenous fluids administered. Multiple risk factors may contribute to wound healing complications, and the decision to transfuse is made on an individual case basis according to symptoms and other patient-specific factors. In this study, data on intraoperative estimated blood loss were not collected owing to the potential for imprecise measurement and subjective bias; instead, drain output was selected as a more reliable measure of the patient's propensity to bleed in the perioperative period. Given that drain output averaged 83.3 mL per case lower after preoperative warfarin, a similar reduction in blood loss may have occurred during surgery itself but would not have been detected in this study.

Finally, patient morbidity and mortality owing to pulmonary embolus, which remain the most clinically relevant outcomes, occur so infrequently that they can only be feasibly evaluated in large database studies or metaanalyses. Our study, like the vast majority of the literature on this subject, was not powered to compare the rates of symptomatic DVT, nor was this our goal. Rather, it was intended to evaluate INR, drain output, and change in hemoglobin; therefore, as in most publications, the sample size is too small to determine significant differences in the rates of major adverse events.

SUMMARY

In our study of 165 patients undergoing primary, elective THA or TKA, initiation of warfarin therapy on the night before surgery compared with the night after surgery was associated with significantly decreased drain output and earlier increases in postoperative INR; however, we did not observe a statistically significant difference in perioperative change in hemoglobin. Although we were unable to detect any difference in complication rates between groups, larger studies are needed to more definitively determine whether the risk of adverse events is decreased with either strategy.

REFERENCES

1. Preventing venous thromboembolic disease in patients undergoing elective hip and knee arthroplasty: evidence-based guideline and evidence report. 2nd edition. Rosemont (IL): American Academy of Orthopaedic Surgeons; 2011.

2. Markel DC, York S, Liston MJ Jr, et al, AAHKS Research Committee. Venous thromboembolism: management by American Association of Hip and Knee Surgeons. J Arthroplasty 2010;25(1):3–9.e1-2.

3. Warwick D, Rosencher N. The "critical thrombosis period" in major orthopedic surgery: when to start and when to stop prophylaxis. Clin Appl Thromb Hemost 2010;16(4):394–405.

4. Arcelus JI, Monreal M, Caprini JA, et al. Clinical presentation and time-course of postoperative venous thromboembolism: results from the RIETE Registry. Thromb Haemost 2008;99:546–51.

5. Bjørnarå BT, Gudmundsen TE, Dahl OE. Frequency and timing of clinical venous thromboembolism after major joint surgery. J Bone Joint Surg Br 2006; 88:386–91.

6. Seagroatt V, Tan HS, Goldacre M, et al. Elective total hip replacement: incidence, emergency readmission rate, and postoperative mortality. BMJ 1991;303:1431–5.

7. White RH, Romano PS, Zhou H, et al. Incidence and time course of thromboembolic outcomes following total hip or knee arthroplasty. Arch Intern Med 1998;158:1525–31.

8. Hull RD, Brant RF, Pineo GF, et al. Preoperative vs postoperative initiation of low-molecular-weight heparin prophylaxis against venous thromboembolism in

patients undergoing elective hip replacement. Arch Intern Med 1999;159(2):137–41.

9. Hull RD, Pineo GF, Stein PD, et al. Timing of initial administration of low-molecular-weight heparin prophylaxis against deep vein thrombosis in patients following elective hip arthroplasty: a systematic review [Review]. Arch Intern Med 2001;161(16): 1952–60.

10. Kwong LM, Muntz JE. Thromboprophylaxis dosing: the relationship between timing of first administration, efficacy, and safety [Review]. Am J Orthop (Belle Mead NJ) 2002;31(11 Suppl):16–20.

11. Perka C. Preoperative versus postoperative initiation of thromboprophylaxis following major orthopedic surgery: safety and efficacy of postoperative administration supported by recent trials of new oral anticoagulants. Thromb J 2011;9:17.

12. Raskob GE, Hirsh J. Controversies in timing of the first dose of anticoagulant prophylaxis against venous thromboembolism after major orthopedic surgery [Review]. Chest 2003;124(6 Suppl):379S–85S.

13. Strebel N, Prins M, Agnelli G, et al. Preoperative or postoperative start of prophylaxis for venous thromboembolism with low-molecular-weight heparin in elective hip surgery? [Review]. Arch Intern Med 2002;162(13):1451–6.

14. Tribout B, Colin-Mercier F. New versus established drugs in venous thromboprophylaxis: efficacy and safety considerations related to timing of administration [Review]. Am J Cardiovasc Drugs 2007;7(1): 1–15.

15. Esmon CT, Vigano-D'Angelo S, D'Angelo A, et al. Anticoagulation proteins C and S [Review]. Adv Exp Med Biol 1987;214:47–54.

16. Vigano D'Angelo S, Comp PC, Esmon CT, et al. Relationship between protein C antigen and anticoagulant activity during oral anticoagulation and in selected disease states. J Clin Invest 1986;77(2): 416–25.

Impact of Inpatient Versus Outpatient Total Joint Arthroplasty on 30-Day Hospital Readmission Rates and Unplanned Episodes of Care

Bryan D. Springer, MD[a],*, Susan M. Odum, PhD[b],
David N. Vegari, MD[c], Jeffrey G. Mokris, MD[a],
Walter B. Beaver Jr, MD[a]

KEYWORDS

- Total joint arthroplasty • Total knee arthroplasty • Total hip arthroplasty • Hospital readmission

---

KEY POINTS

- With the advent of rapid rehabilitation protocols and improved perioperative pain management, total joint arthroplasty (TJA) is rapidly moving toward shorter hospital length of stay (LOS) and outpatient TJA.
- The purpose of this study was to compare hospital LOS 30-day readmissions, all unplanned care episodes, and patient satisfaction between outpatient and inpatient TJA.
- Although not statistically significant, this study showed a higher rate of unplanned 30-day hospital readmissions following outpatient TJA (11.7%) than inpatient TJA (6.6%).
- A significantly higher proportion of patients who had an outpatient TJA reported that they received excellent care the day of their surgery.

INTRODUCTION

It is estimated that the number of total hip and knee arthroplasties (THA and TKA, respectively) will double within the next decade.[1] The economic burden associated with this projected increased demand may be astronomical. Health care entities must decrease costs as total joint arthroplasty (TJA) utilization increases. One potential way to curb hospital costs is by minimizing patients' hospital length of stay (LOS). Studies from the mid-1990s showed that LOS can be reduced (from 6.79 to 4.16 days) without affecting patient outcomes.[2] With recent advances in pain management, rehabilitation, and protocol-driven treatment, outpatient TJA is becoming more popular.[3,4]

With the passage of the Patient Protection and Affordable Care Act in 2010, there has been increased focus on health care savings. The federal government has a keen interest in unplanned readmissions of patients within 30 days from surgery. If a hospital's readmission rate exceeded the Center for Medicare and Medicaid Services (CMS) parameters, then hospitals were penalized 1% of total revenues in 2013. This number rose to 2% in 2014 and 3%

Disclosure Statement: There was no external funding source. None of the authors have a proprietary interest in the materials described in this article.
[a] OrthoCarolina Hip & Knee Center, 2001 Vail Avenue, Suite 200A, Charlotte, NC 28207, USA; [b] OrthoCarolina Research Institute, 2001 Vail Avenue, Suite 300, Charlotte, NC 28207, USA; [c] Lankenau Medical Center, Lankenau MOB East, 100 East Lancaster Avenue, Suite 256, Wynnewood, PA 19096, USA
* Corresponding author.
E-mail address: Bryan.Springer@orthocarolina.com

in 2015. CMS parameters are based on national averages adjusted for various hospitalizations and procedures that occur in Inpatient Prospective Payment System (IPPS) hospitals. In 2013, the penalties were linked only to those readmissions associated with an underlying diagnosis of myocardial infarction, pneumonia, or congestive heart failure. However, CMS proposed to add chronic obstructive pulmonary disease and TJA, with a potential 3% penalty for 2015.

Several reports in the literature have shown that a successful outpatient TJA can be accomplished; however, many fail to consider readmission rates. As hospitals aim to decrease LOS concurrent with pending significant financial penalties for unplanned readmissions, one must closely assess the impact that hospital LOS might have on unplanned hospital readmissions. As the insurance industry looks toward a bundled payment arrangement with hospitals, unplanned care episodes that do not result in a hospital readmission, such as emergency room (ER) visits, also become important. The purpose of this study was to compare 30-day hospital readmission rates for patients undergoing outpatient and inpatient TJA and determine if LOS impacted hospital readmission rates and unplanned care episodes.

PATIENTS AND METHODS

In September 2010, 1 arthroplasty surgeon at the authors' institution developed a clinical pathway to perform outpatient primary TJA. In order to potentially qualify for outpatient arthroplasty, several preoperative criteria had to be met:

1. Healthy patients with no active cardiopulmonary conditions
2. No history of sleep apnea, deep venous thrombosis, or pulmonary embolus
3. Must live within 1 hour of the hospital where index procedure was performed
4. Must have good family support at home
5. Body mass index (BMI) less than 40

Between September 2010 and May 2011, the authors retrospectively reviewed the charts of patients who had undergone outpatient (same day discharge to home) TJA. The same inclusion criteria were used to retrospectively identify a separate cohort of patients who had undergone a TJA at the same hospital during the same time period by 2 other surgeons. These patients met the criteria for outpatient TJA but were admitted for an LOS of at least 2 days based on surgeon's judgment.

A review of all patients' electronic medical records was undertaken to determine unplanned hospital readmissions, urgent care or ER visits, or other complications during the 30-day postoperative period. Each patient was contacted via telephone to determine any additional readmissions or unplanned care visits related to their surgery. Patients were also polled regarding their satisfaction with their surgery and hospital stay.

Statistical analysis was performed using SAS Version 9.2 (SAS Institute Incorporated, Cary, North Carolina). Standard descriptive statistics including frequency, proportions, means, and variation are reported. The dependent variable for all differential analyses was readmission as a binary variable. A chi-square test was used to determine differences in proportions. An independent t-test was used to determine statistical differences in the mean patient age and BMI at the time of surgery between those who had a TJA as an inpatient procedure and those who had an outpatient TJA. An alpha level of significance of 0.05 was used to determine statistical significance for all tests.

Between September 2010 and May 2011, 232 patients underwent an outpatient TJA procedure. Of the 232 outpatient TJA patients, 42 (18%) patients required an overnight hospital stay and were excluded from further analyses. Table 1 lists the reasons why these planned outpatient TJAs required overnight admission, as well as 30-day readmission details. Of the remaining 190 outpatient TJA patients, 53 (28%) were not available to complete the phone survey and were considered lost to follow-up. Therefore, 137 of the 190 (72%) outpatient TJA patients were included in the final analyses. During the same time period, 148 patients underwent inpatient TJA with a minimum 2-day hospital stay. Of the 148 patients, 106 patients (70.9%) completed the telephone survey. The study population consisted of 243 patients (137 outpatients and 106 inpatients). Table 2 reports the demographics of both study groups.

Of the 243 patients included in the study, 166 underwent primary TKA, and 77 underwent primary THA. All inpatient and outpatient TKAs were performed using spinal or general anesthesia, a medial parapatellar approach, and included perioperative multimodal pain management. All inpatient and outpatient THAs were performed under spinal or general anesthesia at the discretion of the anesthesiologist. A standard posterior lateral approach and included perioperative multimodal pain management, which included nonsteroidal

Table 1
Reason for staying

Patient Number	Age	Gender	Procedure	Body Mass Index	Reason for Staying	30-Day Readmission
1	53	F	THA	32.3	Low blood pressure	N
2	70	M	TKA	32.6	Unresolved spinal	N
3	60	F	TKA	33.7	Weakness	N
4	57	M	THA	33.8	Late surgery	N
5	47	M	THA	34	Low blood pressure	N
6	73	M	THA	38.6	Inadequate pain control	N
7	53	F	TKA	40	Low oxygen	N
8	64	F	TKA	39.9	Inadequate pain control	N
9	67	M	TKA	40.6	Inadequate pain control	N
10	56	F	TKA	40.6	Inadequate pain control	N
11	69	F	TKA	42.9	Patient refused discharge	N
12	66	F	TKA	43.4	Unresolved spinal	N
13	53	F	TKA	36.2	Inadequate pain control	N
14	82	F	THA	19.8	Weakness	N
15	47	F	TKA	22.3	Inadequate pain control	N
16	74	F	TKA	23.9	Low blood pressure	N
17	55	F	THA	24.1	Weakness	Y: Hospital-PE
18	58	F	TKA	26.1	Low blood pressure	N
19	45	M	THA	26.3	Low blood pressure	Y: Hospital-MRSA Infection
20	47	F	TKA	26.3	Nausea/vomiting	N
21	54	M	THA	26.4	Low blood pressure	N
22	53	F	THA	26.5	Weakness	N
23	53	F	THA	26.5	Nausea/vomiting	N
24	45	M	THA	26.6	Unresolved spinal	N
25	72	F	TKA	26.6	Weakness	N
26	83	M	TKA	26.7	Low Blood Pressure	N
27	45	M	THA	26.7	Unresolved Spinal	N
28	80	M	TKA	26.9	Low blood pressure	N
29	61	M	THA	27.6	Home care not arranged	N
30	87	F	TKA	27.9	Weakness	N
31	59	M	TKA	28.9	Inadequate pain control	N
32	65	M	THA	31.4	Unresolved spinal	N
33	66	F	THA	25.2	Inadequate pain control	N
34	55	F	TKA	38.8	Inadequate pain control	N
35	60	F	TKA	44.3	Inadequate pain control	N
36	64	M	THA	30	Weakness	N
37	62	F	TKA	24.9	Nausea/vomiting	N
38	65	M	TKA	28.4	Patient refused discharge	N
39	46	F	TKA	33.1	Inadequate pain control	N
40	69	F	TKA	33.8	Nausea/vomiting	N
41	69	F	THA	28.7	Low blood pressure	N
42	75	F	THA	21.5	Low blood pressure	N

Table 2
Demographics

Variable	Inpatient	Outpatient	P Value
Age (years)	65	61	.0008
BMI	20	31	<.0001
Follow-up (months)	28	10	<.0001
Ranges			
Age (years)	39–87	28–84	—
BMI	19–28	19–54	—
Follow-up (months)	24–34	5–16	—
Gender			
Female	61 (57.55%)	60 (43.80%)	.0335
Male	45 (42.45%)	77 (56.20%)	—

anti-inflammatories, oral acetaminophen, short-acting oral narcotics, and either local periarticular joint injection or peripheral nerve blocks were utilized. **Fig. 1** illustrates the breakdown of the study sample.

RESULTS
30-Day Hospital Readmissions
Overall, there were 18 (7.4%) unplanned hospital readmissions within 30 days of surgery in both groups. Of the 137 outpatient TJA procedures, 12 patients (8.8%) were readmitted within 30 days, while 6 of 106 inpatient TJAs (5.7%) required hospital readmission within 30 days. With the available sample size, this difference was not statistically significant ($P = .36$). When evaluating early readmissions, 9 outpatients (6.6%) required readmission within the first 4 days after discharge compared with 4 patients (3.8%) in the inpatient cohort ($P = .25$). A complete list of the reasons for hospital readmission is reported in **Table 3**.

30-Day Readmissions by Procedure Type
Of the 166 TKA patients, 18 (11%) required readmission. No THA patients (inpatient or outpatient) required a 30-day hospital readmission. This difference was statistically significant ($P = .0011$). In the outpatient TKA cohort, 12 patients (13%) had a hospital readmission, compared with 6 patients (8%) in the inpatient TKA group ($P = .31$). **Fig. 1** illustrates the number of hospital readmissions and unplanned care episodes stratified by procedure type.

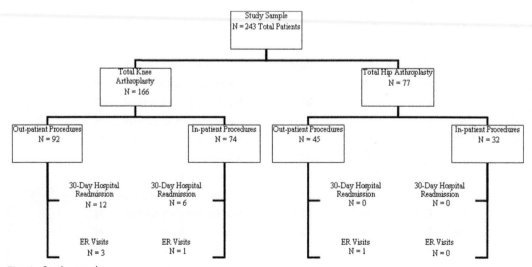

Fig. 1. Study sample.

Table 3
Readmission reasons

Patient Number	Group	30-Day Readmission	Episode of Care	Reason for Readmission
1	Outpatient	Y	Hospital readmission	Adverse reaction to pain medication
2	Outpatient	Y	Hospital readmission	Infection
3	Outpatient	Y	Hospital readmission	Wound complication
4	Outpatient	Y	Hospital readmission	Pain pump failure (pain)
5	Outpatient	Y	Hospital readmission	Low O_2, Anemia
6	Outpatient	Y	Hospital readmission	Adverse reaction to pain medication
7	Outpatient	Y	Hospital readmission	Adverse reaction to pain medication
8	Outpatient	Y	Urgent care	Adverse reaction to pain medication
9	Outpatient	Y	Hospital readmission	Wound complication
10	Outpatient	N	Emergency room	Wound complication
11	Outpatient	Y	Hospital readmission	Wound complication
12	Outpatient	N	Emergency room	Inadequate pain control
13	Outpatient	Y	Hospital readmission	Pain pump failure (pain)
14	Outpatient	Y	Hospital readmission	Pain pump failure (pain)
15	Outpatient	N	Emergency room	Adverse reaction to pain medication
16	Outpatient	N	Emergency room	Excessive pain and swelling
1	Inpatient	Y	Hospital readmission	Wound complication
2	Inpatient	Y	Hospital readmission	Skin rash (non wound)
3	Inpatient	Y	Hospital readmission	Inadequate pain control
4	Inpatient	Y	Hospital readmission	Excessive swelling
5	Inpatient	Y	Hospital readmission	Excessive fatigue
6	Inpatient	Y	Hospital readmission	Wound complication
7	Inpatient	N	Emergency Room	Inadequate pain control

30-Day Readmissions Plus Unplanned Care Episodes

When including unplanned care episodes that did not require full admission to the hospital (ER visits and urgent care visits) for TKA and THA procedures combined, 16 (11.7%) outpatients required either hospital readmission or unplanned care episode compared with 7 (6.6%) inpatients. One inpatient surgical procedure (TKA) patient and 4 outpatient surgical procedure (3 TKA +1 THA) patients had an unplanned nonadmission episode of care in an ER or urgent care center. With the available sample size, this difference was not statistically significant ($P = .18$). When stratified by procedure type, 22 TKA patients (13%) required either a hospital readmission or unplanned episode of care, compared with 1 THA patient (1.2%) who required an unplanned visit to the ER ($P = .0018$).

Patient Satisfaction

Patients completed a telephone survey that consisted of 15 individual survey questions, and 7 of these were selected as specific measures of patient satisfaction. Table 4 presents the proportions of the 5 possible patient responses to each of the satisfaction questions for each group. To compare the differences in satisfaction between patients who underwent an inpatient TJA and patients who had an outpatient total joint, the 5 responses were collapsed into 2 categories. Only the highest rating responses (eg, excellent or strongly agree) were defined as satisfied, while all other responses were considered not satisfied. There was no significant difference between groups with patients' desire to recommend the respective procedure to friends and family (80% inpatient, 71% outpatient, $P = .25$). Eighty-six percent of the patients in the inpatient group and 91% of patients in the

Table 4 Patient satisfaction data					
Level of care that patients received at the hospital the day of surgery					
	Excellent	**Above average**	**Average**	**Below average**	**Poor**
Inpatient	87 (82)	14 (13)	2 (2)	1 (1)	2 (2)
Outpatient	128 (93)	6 (4)	2 (2)	0 (0)	1 (1)
Recommend this procedure to friends and family					
	Strongly agree	**Agree**	**Neither**	**Disagree**	**Strongly disagree**
Inpatient	82 (80)	19 (18)	1 (1)	1 (1)	0 (0)
Outpatient	97 (71)	32 (23)	3 (2)	2 (1)	3 (2)
Frequency missing = 3					
Overall satisfaction with the procedure with respect to friendliness of the staff					
	Excellent	**Above average**	**Average**	**Below average**	**Poor**
Inpatient	90 (86)	9 (8)	4 (4)	1 (1)	1 (1)
Outpatient	125 (91)	10 (7)	2 (2)	0 (0)	0 (0)
Frequency missing = 1					
Overall satisfaction based on the surgeon's information about what to expect from the surgical procedure is					
	Excellent	**Above average**	**Average**	**Below average**	**Poor**
Inpatient	82 (78)	17 (16)	5 (5)	1 (1)	0 (0)
Outpatient	107 (78)	19 (14)	6 (4)	3 (2)	2 (2)
Frequency missing = 1					
Overall satisfaction based on the surgeon's information about what to expect from my recovery at home is					
	Excellent	**Above average**	**Average**	**Below average**	**Poor**
Inpatient	73 (69)	21 (20)	8 (8)	3 (3)	0 (0)
Outpatient	103 (75)	16 (12)	11 (8)	6 (4)	1 (1)
Frequency missing = 1					
Overall satisfaction with the procedure with respect to the capability of the surgeon is					
	Excellent	**Above average**	**Average**	**Below average**	**Poor**
Inpatient	95 (90)	6 (6)	4 (4)	0 (0)	0 (0)
Outpatient	123 (90)	12 (9)	1 (<1)	1 (<1)	0 (0)
Frequency missing = 1					
Overall satisfaction with the procedure with respect to an improvement in my quality of life is					
	Excellent	**Above average**	**Average**	**Below average**	**Poor**
Inpatient	64 (61)	27 (26)	10 (9)	3 (3)	1 (1)
Outpatient	88 (64)	28 (20)	13 (10)	2 (2)	6 (4)
Frequency missing = 1					

outpatient group (P = .13) were satisfied with the friendliness of the hospital staff. Most patients in the study regardless of procedure type were satisfied with the expectation of the surgery (P = .89) and the expectation of the recovery period from surgery (P = .28) as set forth by the surgeon. Ninety percent of patients in

each group (P = .97) were satisfied with the capability of the surgeon. Finally, most inpatient TJA patients (61%) and outpatient TJA patients (64%) were satisfied with the quality of life achieved following surgery. A significantly (P = .006) higher proportion of patients who had an outpatient TJA reported that they received excellent care the day of their surgery. Of the 106 inpatient TJA patients, 87 (82%) reported the care received the day of surgery as excellent compared with 93% (128 of 137) of those patients who underwent outpatient TJA.

DISCUSSION

With the advent of rapid rehabilitation protocols and improved perioperative pain management, TJA is rapidly moving toward shorter hospital LOS and outpatient TJA.[4–8] The implementation of the Patient Care and Affordability Act has created increased scrutiny of 30-day hospital readmissions. Beginning in 2015, TJA was included in this scrutiny, with the potential for 3% penalties of total hospital reimbursements from CMS. Clement and colleagues[9] determined that if Medicare stopped reimbursing for readmission after THA, their hospital would lose $11,494 per episode of care that required readmission.

Additionally, hospital reimbursement and public reporting of quality will be tied to patient satisfaction. At potential odds with this is a desire to cut costs by reducing hospital LOS. The purpose of our study was to compare hospital LOS 30-day readmissions, all unplanned care episodes, and patient satisfaction between outpatient and inpatient TJA.

This study has several strengths and limitations. In an attempt to minimize selection bias, the authors conducted an exhaustive chart review to select a sample of inpatient, 2-day LOS, using the same medical criteria used for outpatient procedure appropriateness:

- Healthy patients with no active cardiopulmonary conditions
- No history of sleep apnea, deep venous thrombosis, or pulmonary embolus
- Must live within 1 hour of the hospital where index procedure was performed
- Must have good family support at home
- BMI less than 40

However, it was not possible to derive an exact match for the entire group such as type of anesthesia utilized. Surgeries were performed at a single institution, using similar perioperative protocols. Thirty-day readmissions and patient satisfaction scores were subsequently obtained via telephone conversations and statistically analyzed to determine significance. This study is limited by the retrospective nature, relatively large lost-to-follow-up (28%) and relatively small sample size (N = 243). A total of 425 per group is needed to find a significant difference with

80% power with these results (6.6% inpatient vs 11.7% outpatient readmissions). In addition to a search of the Social Security Death Index, the authors conducted patient telephone interviews to increase follow-up and obtain patient satisfaction data. Recall bias is an inherent factor, and patient recollection may be insufficient to key details associated with all unplanned care for which the authors do not have access. Thus these numbers most likely represent the best case scenario for hospital readmission and unplanned care episodes. If one assumed that all patients lost to follow-up were readmitted within 30 days, the readmission rate would be 34% (65 of 190) for outpatient TJA patients and 32% (48 of 149) for inpatient TJA patients ($P = .39$).

Multiple studies have investigated readmission rates as a factor of LOS for inpatient TJA.[10,11] None, however, have specifically compared inpatient versus outpatient TJA. Although not statistically significant, the authors' study showed a higher rate of unplanned 30-day hospital readmissions following outpatient TJA (11.7%) than inpatient TJA (6.6%). This was particularly true for patients undergoing outpatient TKA, where the readmission rates were double (12% vs 6%) those of inpatient TKA.

The higher readmission rate for same-day procedures mirrors a similarly matched inpatient cohort reported with CMS data. Lovald and colleagues[12] found a 2.18 hazard ratio for 90-day readmission for outpatient and short LOS TKA compared with their standard stay of 3 to 4 days. However, this was not statistically significant.

Berger and colleagues have reported extensively on their experience with same-day discharge after TKA. Their initial results demonstrated comparable readmission rates to those that the authors found. In 86 outpatient TKAs, 5 patients (5.8%) were either readmitted or visited the ER (4 readmissions and 1 ER visit) during the first week.[3,4,13] Over the first 3 months following outpatient TKA, an additional 4 readmissions and 1 emergency visit took place (11.6%).[13] These data was not stratified to assess 30-day readmission, nor was there a comparative inpatient cohort. Kolisek and colleagues[14] found no difference in readmission rates or complication rates between their same-day and overnight TKA cohorts. The authors' data did demonstrate a statistically significant difference in readmission rates between TKA and THA patients. No THA patients in the authors' study, inpatient or outpatient, had a 30-day hospital readmission, and only 1 patient had an unplanned episode of care (ER visit). This lower readmission rate for THA seems to be consistent with other studies on readmission rates with reduced LOS for outpatient THA.

Dorr's study of readmission rates for same-day hip surgery is comparable to the authors' experience regarding readmission rates for same-day THA.[15] His group found that 53 patients (100%) at 6 month following their operations had no readmissions for medical complications. There was 1 readmission (1.9%) for an unrecognized intraoperative calcar fracture that necessitated femoral component revision.

Patient satisfaction is becoming an increasingly important metric used by hospitals and payers. It will ultimately be tied to reimbursement and pay for performance for both hospitals and physicians. The data on patient satisfaction following outpatient TJA are relatively sparse. In the authors' study, patients were equally satisfied with both inpatient and outpatient TJA, as measured by 13 metrics. This finding is consistent with Dorr's outpatient THA study that found 96% of patients were satisfied with the decision to have outpatient surgery.[15] Similarly, Mont's study on outpatient versus inpatient TKA found no difference in mean satisfaction scores between the 2 cohorts.[14]

In order to facilitate a reduction in readmission rates following TJA, one must identify those patients who are at higher risk for readmission preoperatively as well as understand the etiology of readmissions. Several recent studies have evaluated risk factors for hospital readmission following TJA. The most common risk factors reported include increasing age, obesity, diabetes, coronary artery disease, high American Society of Anesthesiologists physical status score, and elevated blood urea nitrogen levels.[12,16–19] The authors' outpatient treatment guidelines define patients with BMI greater than 40, active cardiopulmonary disease, a history of sleep apnea, or a history of venous thromboembolic events as high risk, and they are not outpatient surgical candidates. As a result, the authors had few readmissions for medical reasons. In the authors' study population, most hospital readmissions and unplanned care episodes were associated with inadequate pain control, intolerance of pain medications, and wound complications care episodes. These findings are consistent with multiple studies reporting that wound complications, wound infections, and pain are leading causes of hospital readmissions and unplanned care episodes following TJA.[9,16,18,20,21]

SUMMARY

Thirty-day hospital readmission was higher for TKA than for THA, regardless of patient disposition. Although not statistically significant, readmissions for TKAs performed on an outpatient basis were almost double that for TKAs with a 2-day LOS. This may have financial implications to hospitals in the form of penalties for increased readmission rates as well as bundled care arrangements for unplanned care episodes. These financial penalties for unplanned readmission must be weighed against the benefits and potential cost savings of outpatient TJA. Improved perioperative protocols, patient education, and clinical care pathways designed specifically for outpatient TJA should help lower the overall rate of hospital readmissions and unplanned care episodes.

REFERENCES

1. Fehring TK, Odum SM, Troyer JL, et al. Joint replacement access in 2016: a supply side crisis. J Arthroplasty 2010;25(8):1175–81.
2. Healy WL, Iorio R, Ko J, et al. Impact of cost reduction programs on short-term patient outcome and hospital cost of total knee arthroplasty. J Bone Joint Surg Am 2002;84-A(3):348–53.
3. Berger RA. A comprehensive approach to outpatient total hip arthroplasty. Am J Orthop (Belle Mead NJ) 2007;36(9 Suppl):4–5.
4. Berger RA, Sanders SA, Thill ES, et al. Newer anesthesia and rehabilitation protocols enable outpatient hip replacement in selected patients. Clin Orthop Relat Res 2009;467(6):1424–30.
5. Berend KR, Lombardi AV Jr, Mallory TH. Rapid recovery protocol for peri-operative care of total hip and total knee arthroplasty patients. Surg Technol Int 2004;13:239–47.
6. Berger RA, Jacobs JJ, Meneghini RM, et al. Rapid rehabilitation and recovery with minimally invasive total hip arthroplasty. Clin Orthop Relat Res 2004;(429):239–47.
7. Healy WL, Ayers ME, Iorio R, et al. Impact of a clinical pathway and implant standardization on total hip arthroplasty: a clinical and economic study of short-term patient outcome. J Arthroplasty 1998; 13(3):266–76.
8. Peters CL, Shirley B, Erickson J. The effect of a new multimodal perioperative anesthetic regimen on postoperative pain, side effects, rehabilitation, and length of hospital stay after total joint arthroplasty. J Arthroplasty 2006;21(6 Suppl 2):132–8.
9. Clement RC, Derman PB, Graham DS, et al. Risk factors, causes, and the economic implications of

unplanned readmissions following total hip arthroplasty. J Arthroplasty 2013;28(8 Suppl):7–10.

10. Cram P, Lu X, Kates SL, et al. Total knee arthroplasty volume, utilization, and outcomes among Medicare beneficiaries, 1991-2010. JAMA 2012; 308(12):1227–36.

11. Wolf BR, Lu X, Li Y, et al. Adverse outcomes in hip arthroplasty: long-term trends. J Bone Joint Surg Am 2012;94(14):e103.

12. Lovald ST, Ong KL, Malkani AL, et al. Complications, mortality, and costs for outpatient and short-stay total knee arthroplasty patients in comparison to standard-stay patients. J Arthroplasty 2014;29(3):510–5.

13. Berger RA, Sanders S, D'Ambrogio E, et al. Minimally invasive quadriceps-sparing TKA: results of a comprehensive pathway for outpatient TKA. J Knee Surg 2006;19(2):145–8.

14. Kolisek FR, McGrath MS, Jessup NM, et al. Comparison of outpatient versus inpatient total knee arthroplasty. Clin Orthop Relat Res 2009;467(6): 1438–42.

15. Dorr LD, Thomas DJ, Zhu J, et al. Outpatient total hip arthroplasty. J Arthroplasty 2010;25(4):501–6.

16. Avram V, Petruccelli D, Winemaker M, et al. Total joint arthroplasty readmission rates and reasons for 30-day hospital readmission. J Arthroplasty 2014;29(3):465–8.

17. Mesko NW, Bachmann KR, Kovacevic D, et al. Thirty-day readmission following total hip and knee arthroplasty - a preliminary single institution predictive model. J Arthroplasty 2014;29(8):1532–8.

18. Saucedo JM, Marecek GS, Wanke TR, et al. Understanding readmission after primary total hip and knee arthroplasty: who's at risk? J Arthroplasty 2014;29(2):256–60.

19. Schairer WW, Sing DC, Vail TP, et al. Causes and frequency of unplanned hospital readmission after total hip arthroplasty. Clin Orthop Relat Res 2014; 472(2):464–70.

20. Bohm ER, Dunbar MJ, Frood JJ, et al. Rehospitalizations, early revisions, infections, and hospital resource use in the first year after hip and knee arthroplasties. J Arthroplasty 2012;27(2):232–7.e1.

21. Vorhies JS, Wang Y, Herndon J, et al. Readmission and length of stay after total hip arthroplasty in a national Medicare sample. J Arthroplasty 2011; 26(6 Suppl):119–23.

Trauma

Timing of Operative Debridement in Open Fractures

Joshua C. Rozell, MD[a,b], Keith P. Connolly, MD[a,b],
Samir Mehta, MD[b],*

KEYWORDS

• Open fracture • Debridement • Surgical timing • Antibiotics

KEY POINTS

- Patients with open fractures are at high risk of infection if not treated expediently.
- The historic 6-hour time limit for debridement of open fractures has been challenged in contemporary publications.
- In the context of early antibiotic administration, debridement within 6 hours has not been shown to be an independent risk factor for infection after open fracture.
- Delayed versus primary wound closure is determined based on the clinical experience of the surgeon, but may not have an effect on infection rates.

BACKGROUND

An open fracture is defined as a fracture that involves a violation of the soft tissue envelope with communication through to the fracture fragments, the associated fracture hematoma, or both.[1] Although Gustilo and Anderson[2] espoused universal agreement that open fractures require emergent treatment to include adequate irrigation and surgical debridement of the open wound, few issues in orthopedics today are debated more than the appropriate timing and management of open fractures.[3–11] However, there is consensus that these low- or high-energy injuries result in wound contamination, devitalized tissue, local edema, and surrounding ischemia that interfere with the body's natural immune defense mechanisms to resist infection.[12] As a result of thorough surgical techniques, antibiotic options and administration, and advanced techniques for soft tissue coverage, the ability to manage open fractures has improved. The treating orthopedic surgeon must be able to address these injuries appropriately to limit the risk of infection and promote adequate healing.

This article addresses the evaluation of a patient with an open fracture and analyzes the evidentiary support regarding the historic "6-hour rule" in the timing of operative management.

HISTORICAL PERSPECTIVE

The use of excisional debridement to prevent wound infection dates back to the time of Hippocrates.[13] In 1898, a German military surgeon and bacteriologist, Paul Leopold Friedrich, conducted an experiment using guinea pigs whereby he created open wounds in the triceps region and contaminated them with mud and house dust. Wounds were cleaned in intervals of 30 minutes. He found that when wounds were debrided within 6 hours of inoculation, the guinea pigs survived. All of the guinea pigs whose wounds were debrided after 8.5 hours died. Thus, Friedrich showed that the early phases of bacterial growth within contaminated

Disclosures: All authors have nothing to disclose.
[a] Department of Orthopaedic Surgery, University of Pennsylvania, Philadelphia, PA, USA; [b] Department of Orthopaedic Surgery, University of Pennsylvania, 3737 Market Street, 6th Floor, Philadelphia, PA 19104, USA
* Corresponding author.
E-mail address: Samir.mehta@uphs.upenn.edu

wounds terminated within 6 to 8 hours after inoculation and that extensive debridement to viable tissue within this time period could decrease the risk of infection.[14–16] Of note, Friedrich's work did not involve administration of local or systemic antibiotics. Before World War II, open injuries were left to heal by secondary intention.[17,18] Military surgeon Joseph Trueta aptly described treatment of an open wound (ie, soft tissue injury) as the principal part of the treatment of an open fracture. He believed that the greatest danger of infection lay not in the infection of the bone, but rather the muscle. By the end of the war, Friedrich's study was adopted to reflect the time required to close open wounds.[14] This "6-hour rule," although based primarily on historical opinion and limited clinical evidence,[11] has since been extrapolated to open fractures and was adopted as a treatment guideline in the orthopedic community for many years.[9,19,20] Not until recently have many studies started to challenge the 6-hour rule, shifting away from the previous doctrine of emergently operating on open fractures.[21]

EPIDEMIOLOGY

The tibia is the most common location for an open fracture.[1] Its proximity to the skin and limited soft tissue envelope enable even low-energy fractures to violate the soft tissue envelope.[6,22] Most open fractures occur in the fifth decade of life, commonly as a result traffic accidents, crush injuries, or falls.[23,24] As with most fracture patterns, there is a bimodal distribution: lower energy injuries occur in the elderly most commonly from falls, whereas higher energy injuries occur in younger patients.[24] In a recent review, Court-Brown and colleagues[25] evaluated the epidemiology of open fractures over a 15-year period. They reported 30.7 open fractures per 100,000 person-years, a steady increase as compared with previous reports of 11.5 per 100,000 person-years.[15,24] In their cohort, 69.1% occurred in males and 30.9% occurred in females.

As a result of the disruption of the protective skin barrier, injuries with exposed bone and soft tissue are more prone to infection. For open tibia fractures, an infection rate of 13% to 25% has been reported.[10] Further studies have elucidated the differences in infection rate based on the Gustilo-Anderson classification system[2,26] and the timing of operative debridement.[6,11,27,28] In a retrospective review by Templeman and colleagues,[29] none of 29 type I fractures, 1 of 36 (3%) type II fractures, and 14 of 68 (21%) type III fractures became infected. Early administration

of antibiotics has been shown to be an extremely important factor in the prevention of infection following open fractures. Although antibiotic administration has been deemed "prophylactic," work by several authors has shown that antibiotic use is actually therapeutic.[30,31] Most current recommendations suggest that antibiotics should be administered for 24 to 48 hours after the last debridement.[5,11,18,21,32]

CLASSIFICATION

The Gustilo-Anderson classification of open fractures is the most commonly used system in current practice.[33] This system takes into consideration the energy of the fracture, soft tissue damage, and the degree of contamination.[34] In their retrospective (n = 673) and prospective (n = 352) reviews of 1052 open fractures,[2] a type I injury was defined as a low-energy injury with minimum soft tissue damage and a small (<1 cm) wound. These were typically inside-out puncture injuries with minimal comminution. A type II injury described a low- to moderate-energy injury with moderate soft tissue damage and an open wound up to 10 cm, but without periosteal stripping. Originally, a type III injury was an umbrella category for either an open, segmental fracture with extensive soft tissue damage, or a traumatic amputation. This description was found to be too inclusive, so Gustilo and colleagues[26] modified their type III classification several years later. A type IIIA injury has adequate soft tissue coverage despite the high-energy comminution and segmental nature, irrespective of the wound size. However, an injury with a wound greater than 10 cm was also characterized as IIIA. A type IIIB open fracture necessitates local or distant flap coverage of areas of exposed bone (not including skin grafting). In addition, these fractures are commonly associated with extensive periosteal stripping (Fig. 1). Finally, a type IIIC injury results in a vascular injury that requires repair to preserve limb survival. Isolated injuries to the anterior or posterior tibial artery are not included in this description (Table 1). Importantly, the final classification of the injury is determined in the operating room.[34] To test the reliability of this system, 245 surgeons were given clinical histories, physical examinations, radiographs, and video footage of the operative debridement of 12 open fractures. The overall interobserver agreement was a moderate 60% (range, 42%–94%).[35]

More recently, the Orthopedic Trauma Association developed a more comprehensive

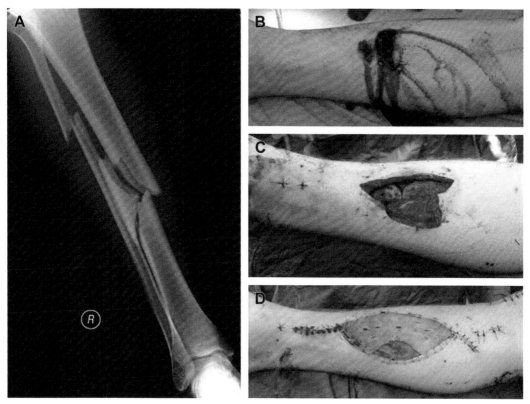

Fig. 1. Anteroposterior radiograph (A) and clinical image (B) of the right tibia in a 27-year-old male who sustained a Gustilo-Anderson type IIIB fracture after a motor vehicle accident. (C) Soft tissue defect after operative debridement. (D) Delayed soft tissue coverage with a rotational soleus flap and split thickness skin grafting. (*Courtesy of* [D] S. Kovach, MD, Philadelphia, PA.)

Table 1 Gustilo-Anderson classification of open fractures	
Subtype	**Description**
I	Wound <1 cm; clean; simple fracture pattern; minimal comminution; minimal soft tissue damage
II	Wound 1–10 cm; simple fracture pattern; moderate soft tissue injury
IIIA	Wound >10 cm; extensive soft tissue injury with maintained soft tissue coverage over bone; high energy, comminuted, or segmental injuries
IIIB	Extensive soft tissue damage with periosteal stripping; inadequate soft tissue coverage of the area of injury
IIIC	Vascular injury requiring repair

Adapted from Cross WW, Swiontkowski MF. Treatment principles in the management of open fractures. Indian J Orthop 2008;42(4):381; with permission.

classification of open fractures, because the Gustilo Anderson classification was designed only for tibial shaft fractures and was shown to have only moderate interobserver reliability.[35] Therefore, based on an extensive review of the literature, the workgroup ranked 34 factors to classify open fractures independent of body site and age. The highest ranking factors included the presence of a skin defect, muscle injury, arterial injury, bone loss, and wound contamination. Contamination was included for its overall contribution to the risk of infection. These factors were each divided into 3 subcategories based on severity. The system was then applied to prospectively collected data of 99 open fractures to determine the clinical feasibility. To accurately assess the zone of injury and the tissue damage, the classification was implemented after the initial operative debridement (Table 2).[36] Although this system represents a comprehensive method to classify open fractures, further study is warranted to evaluate its reliability and validity on a larger scale.

Table 2 Orthopedic trauma association classification of open fractures	
Category	**Severity**
Skin	1. Able to approximate closure 2. Not able to be approximate closure 3. Extensive degloving injury
Muscle	1. No muscle death, intact muscle function 2. Muscle loss but function remains; some necrosis 3. Loss of function, necrotic muscle, disruption of muscle–tendon unit; muscle defect not able to be approximated
Arterial	1. No arterial injury 2. Arterial injury without ischemia 3. Arterial injury with distal ischemia
Contamination	1. None or minimal 2. Superficial contamination 3. (A) Deep contamination; (B) high-risk environment (ie, farm, fecal, dirty water)
Bone loss	1. No bone loss 2. Some bone loss but cortical contact between fragments remains 3. Segmental bone loss

From Orthopedic Trauma Association: Open Fracture Study Group. A new classification scheme for open fractures. J Orthop Trauma 2010;24:460; with permission.

INITIAL MANAGEMENT

The management of an open fracture begins in the emergency department. Antibiotics and tetanus prophylaxis should be administered in a timely fashion as early as possible.[9,21,32,34] Any patient presenting with an open fracture who has not completed the tetanus toxoid immunization series or has not had their booster in the last 5 years should be given a tetanus toxoid booster. If the wound is prone to contamination with *Clostridium tetani*, the tetanus toxoid should be combined with human tetanus immune globulin. If more than 10 years have elapsed since the last tetanus booster or the patient has a compromised immune system, both tetanus toxoid and human tetanus immune globulin should be administered.[34]

After an initial evaluation of the soft tissue injury and neurovascular status, the wound should be covered with a sterile dressing and the limb immobilized in a well-padded splint.[22] The splint will assist in stabilizing the fracture and limit further shear forces across the soft tissue by limiting excessive motion of the bone fragments. Repeated uncovering and covering of the wound has been shown to increase the rate of infection by 3- to 4-fold,[1,37] so a sterile or betadine-soaked[18] dressing should be applied and not removed until the patient is in the operating room. If there is obvious debris or contamination this should be removed and irrigation at the bedside with a gentle normal saline lavage considered, but deeper debridement should be avoided at the risk of further contamination of the tissues with nosocomial organisms.[22]

ANTIBIOTIC ADMINISTRATION

The urgent administration of antibiotics is a well-established critical step in preventing infection of open fractures. A systematic review of antibiotic administration in open fractures by the Eastern Association for the Surgery of Trauma produced several recommendations for treatment. This review found Level 1 evidence for 4 statements:

1. Systemic antibiotic coverage directed at gram-positive organisms should be initiated as soon as possible after injury,
2. Additional gram-negative coverage should be added for type III fractures,
3. High-dose penicillin should be added in the presence of fecal or potential clostridial contamination (eg, farm-related injuries), and
4. Fluoroquinolones offer no advantage compared with cephalosporin/aminoglycoside regimens (Table 3).

Moreover, these agents may have a detrimental effect on fracture healing and may result in higher infection rates in type III open fractures. Additionally, Level 2 recommendations were:

1. In type III fractures, antibiotics should be continued for 72 hours after injury or not greater than 24 hours after soft tissue coverage has been achieved, and
2. Once-daily aminoglycoside dosing is safe and effective for types II and III fractures.[38]

Another recent review of management of open tibial fractures concluded that a first-generation cephalosporin in conjunction with an aminoglycoside is a reasonable antibiotic regimen for type III

Table 3
Recommended antibiotic prophylaxis regimen according to Gustilo-Anderson fracture type

Injury Type	Recommended Antibiotic Prophylaxis
Gustilo-Anderson type I	Systemic first-generation cephalosporin.
Gustilo-Anderson type II	Systemic first-generation cephalosporin.
Gustilo-Anderson Type III	Systemic first-generation cephalosporin plus aminoglycoside. Optional addition of local antibiotic-laden polymethylmethacrylate for large bone or soft tissue defects.
Farm injury or gross soil contamination	Addition of penicillin to above regimen.

open fractures, with the caveat that sufficiently powered randomized trials are still necessary to provide unequivocal evidence.[39] Regarding timing to antibiotic administration, Patzakis and Wilkins[32] previously established that delays of greater than 3 hours resulted in a 1.63 times greater odds of infection compared with those receiving antibiotics less than 3 hours from injury. More recently, a retrospective study found that for type III open tibia fractures, antibiotic administration beyond 66 minutes was independently predictive of infection in multivariate analysis.[40]

The effect of local delivery at the site of wound contamination in open fractures has been the focus of more recent studies on the subject. The utilization of antibiotic-impregnated polymethylmethacrylate cement beads has been shown to be an efficacious tool in the management of open fractures with severe bone or soft tissue defects.[23] Craig and colleagues[41] conducted a metaanalysis of open fractures treated with intramedullary nailing comparing the use of locally delivered antibiotics plus systemic antibiotics with the use of systemic antibiotics alone. They found that the infection rate decreased from 31% for type IIIB and IIIC fractures to 9% for those treated with the addition of locally administered antibiotics. For type IIIA fractures, the rate decreased from 14.4% to 2.4% with the addition of local antibiotics. Included in this review was a retrospective study of 704 open fractures by Osterman and colleagues,[42] which showed an infection rate of 4.2% for those treated with local antibiotics compared with 17% for those treated with systemic antibiotics alone. The available evidence regarding the efficacy of antibiotic-laden cement in large defect open fractures is compelling; however, most studies are of poor quality evidence and larger well-designed comparative studies on the subject are required to better classify the treatment effect accountable to local antibiotic delivery.

TIMING OF DEBRIDEMENT

The effect of delaying debridement beyond the 6-hour time frame is not entirely clear.[43] The pre-antiseptic war era observations and extrapolation of infection risk related to bacterial doubling times were likely contributing factors to development of the 6-hour guideline.[26,44] Three early studies advocated debridement within 6 hours in keeping with the historical perspective.[45–47] Kreder and Armstrong[45] reviewed 56 open tibia fractures in children, reporting that a delay of more than 6 hours was associated with a 25% increased overall infection risk compared with 12% in patients debrided within 6 hours. However, only 8 of the 56 patients were treated after 6 hours of injury, a number too small for statistical analysis of sufficient power. Kindsfater and Jonassen[46] showed a statistically significant difference in the rate of infection for types II and III open tibia fractures debrided beyond 5 hours (38% vs 7%, respectively).

In 1997, the British Orthopedic Association and British Association of Plastic, Reconstructive and Aesthetic Surgeons stated that the first orthopedic debridement procedure should be undertaken within 6 hours of injury.[48] In addition to the notion that deliberately delaying debridement of an open fracture may be unethical, there are a multitude of confounding variables that render a prospective, randomized study on the timing of debridement difficult to implement in a clinical setting.[21] These include surgeon availability, mobilization timing of hospital and operating room resources, and the patient's clinical status. However, over the past 20 years, a large number of studies have sought to investigate and potentially challenge the 6-hour rule, prompting the British Orthopedic Association and the British Association of Plastic, Reconstructive and Aesthetic Surgeons to revise their guidelines in 2009 in favor of debridement within 24 hours of injury. Much of this clinical evidence is derived from retrospective studies suggesting that, with the early administration of antibiotics, surgery may be delayed up to 12 to 24 hours without increasing the risk of infection.[49]

In a rat femur model contaminated with *Staphylococcus aureus* and treated with a 3-day course of a first-generation cephalosporin along with operative debridement, no animal that received antibiotics and surgery 2 hours after injury had detectable bacteria.[48] Extrapolating this time frame to a clinical study, Khatod and colleagues[6] evaluated 106 open fractures and found that there was no increase in infection with respect to patients treated after 6 hours compared with those treated within 6 hours. Further, no infections in any fracture type occurred if the initial operative treatment began within 2 hours of the injury. The overall rate of soft tissue infection was 22.6%, and the incidence of osteomyelitis was 5.7%.[6] Similarly, Tripuraneni and colleagues[27] showed in a retrospective review of 206 patients with open tibia fractures that there was no difference in infectious outcomes based on irrigation and debridement at less than 6 hours (10.8%), 6 to 12 hours (9.5%), and 12 to 24 hours (5.6%). Patients were followed for at least 2 years. Over a 9-year period, Al-Arabi's group included 237 patients in a prospective study of open fracture debridement, citing no significant difference in infection rates for operative management earlier or beyond 6 hours (7.8% vs 9.6%; $P = .64$).[28] They also noted that a delay in antibiotic administration beyond 24 hours was associated with higher infection rates.

Most investigators have limited the evaluation of open fractures to the lower extremity and specifically the tibia given the increased incidence in this location.[20] In a retrospective analysis of 114 open extremity fractures, time delay was not identified as an independent risk factor for the development of deep infection. No difference in the injury-to-operation interval was found between infected patients (5.0 ± 2.0 hours) and uninfected patients (5.7 ± 3.2 hours). Three independent risk factors for fracture infection were identified: higher Gustilo-Anderson type (particularly types IIIB and IIIC), the use of external or internal fixation, and the location of the fracture within the lower leg.[50] By comparison, multiple studies have shown a 0% infection rate in patients with a type I open fracture.[12,29,51–53] Harley's group, in a retrospective review of 215 open fractures, similarly identified increasing fracture severity as a predictor of an higher infection rate. However, a time to debridement of up to

13 hours after injury did not show an increased risk of infection. Univariate logistic regression analysis demonstrated that infection, increasing Gustilo-Anderson type, lower extremity fracture location, mode of fracture fixation, and duration of antibiotic treatment were found to be significantly related to the development of a nonunion.[8]

A recent prospective study of 315 patients with an open extremity fracture analyzed the timing of operative debridement on infection risk. Patients were grouped into categories of 6-hour time intervals and all patients were formally debrided within 24 hours. Type I injuries comprised 22.2%, 29.8% were type II, and there were a total of 48% of type III injuries. All patients received antibiotics. In univariate and multivariate analysis, there was no difference in infection risk between all of the groups up to 1 year after injury. The overall infection risk was 4.4%.[20]

Weber and colleagues[54] used the time to orthopedic intervention to prospectively assess the development of deep infection, but also sought to evaluate the correlation between the timing of antibiotics, Gustilo-Anderson type, fracture location, and transfusion rate on the incidence of deep infection. Overall, 686 subjects completed the 1-year follow-up interview or the 90-day or greater clinical follow-up. Multivariate logistic regression showed no significant association between time to initial debridement and deep infection risk. Because most patients received antibiotics within 3 to 4 hours, there was no correlation between timing of antibiotics and infection risk in this cohort. The more severe injuries (type III) and lower extremity fractures were more likely to develop deep infection (16% and 17%, respectively) compared with type I injuries or upper extremity fractures (1% and 1.5%, respectively). Patients who received a blood transfusion were also more likely to develop a deep infection.[54] These results may help to delineate whether low-grade open fractures and those about the upper extremity require operative debridement emergently (ie, in the middle of the night).

The treatment algorithm for open fractures may also be applied to children. In contrast with Kreder and colleagues' prior study, a large retrospective multicenter review performed by Skaggs and colleagues[13] evaluated 554 open fractures in children 18 years or younger and reported that the infection rates were similar regardless of whether surgery was performed within 6 hours or beyond 7 hours after the injury. The authors note that in the presence of antibiotic therapy, early debridement offers no additional benefit with regard to infection risk. This becomes important for children who need to be referred to tertiary care centers for definitive management of their open fracture.

MULTIPLE DEBRIDEMENTS

In cases of gross wound contamination or a tenuous soft tissue envelope, delayed wound closure allows for multiple debridements and reassessment of the open wound. After the initial debridement, the use of sterile moist dressings, antibiotics beads, or negative pressure wound therapy closure devices can be used temporarily in preparation for further operative management while allowing the egress of bacteria under neutral or negative pressure. Illustrative of the efficacy of negative pressure, in a prospective, randomized study of 25 open fractures comparing standard saline dressings and negative pressure devices, patients in the negative pressure group developed zero acute infections and 2 delayed deep infections, compared with 7 total infections in the standard dressing group.[55]

However, there are no objective clinical guidelines to determine when a wound is amenable to closure and thus the timing of wound closure falls on the experience of the operative surgeon.[51] As such, debate continues regarding the value of immediate versus delayed wound closure in decreasing infection rates.[4,18] Immediate primary closure may decrease patient length of stay, thereby decreasing the incidence of nosocomial infections which account for more infections after open fracture than contamination at the time of injury.[56]

In an early study evaluating delayed versus primary closure for open tibia fractures, Russell and colleagues[4] found that wounds closed primarily after the first debridement had a significantly greater risk of infection compared with wounds closed in a delayed fashion (20% vs 3%, respectively). They supported earlier findings that delayed primary closure at 5 to 7 days after injury is optimal.

In contrast, more recent studies have begun to challenge this approach. Using 6 different wound management techniques, DeLong and colleagues[18] sought to compare the infection and union rates of open fractures. There were 25 type I fractures (21%), 43 type II fractures (36%), 32 type IIIA fractures (27%), 12 type IIIB fractures (10%), and 7 type IIIC fractures (6%) included. Closure methods included immediate primary closure, second-look primary closure, delayed primary closure, delayed skin grafts, delayed flaps, and primary amputation. No differences were found either in union rates or infection rates among the different methods of closure after accounting for injury severity.[18] In light of these results, immediate primary closure may reduce postoperative complications and the potential morbidity associated with repeated operative debridements.

In an effort to form a more objective basis for wound closure, Lenarz and colleagues[51] instituted a protocol for open fracture debridement in which operative cultures were obtained after each washout. The patient was returned to the operating room every 48 hours until cultures were negative before definitive wound closure. If cultures became positive after 48 hours, the patient was observed clinically. For the 248 lower extremity open fractures studied, the mean number of days to closure for type I injuries was 0.76 whereas types IIIB and IIIC injures required a mean of 14.47 and 18.5 days, respectively, to closure. The rate of deep infection was 4.3% and there was overall no difference in infection rate between upper and lower extremity injuries. The low rate of infection, specifically in type III injuries compared with other studies, may be reflected in their multiple debridement protocol. In addition, the presence of a positive culture did not seem to have an effect on the rate of deep infection and wound closure in patients with late positive cultures did not increase the risk of infection. The use of continuous antibiotic therapy during the entire course of treatment up to 6 weeks may have confounded this result, but the authors argue that from a surgical perspective, the best defense against infection is the quality and thoroughness of the surgical debridement.[51]

The ideal irrigant for the washout of open fractures has been investigated thoroughly.[9,39,57,58] In a survey of 984 orthopedic surgeons, there was no consensus on the type of irrigant used and the intensity of lavage for open fracture debridement. The predominant preference, however, was normal saline alone via low-pressure lavage with 3, 6, and 9 L for type I, II, and III fractures, respectively.[23,39,59] Anglen[60] conducted a prospective, randomized study of 400 open fracture patients and found that there was no difference in infection risk if castile soap or bacitracin-impregnated irrigation was used (13% vs 18%, respectively). A significant difference was found, however, in wound healing failure: 4% in the castile soap group and 9.5% in the bacitracin group. This study was followed with a multicenter study including 2447 patient evaluating both the type of irrigant used and the lavage pressure. Patients were followed for

12 months after injury. Reoperation occurred in 13.2% of patients in the high-pressure group and 12.7% of patients in the low-pressure group, which was not significant; reoperation occurred in 14.8% of the castile soap group and 11.6% in the saline group, which was significant. However, with regard to secondary endpoints of nonoperatively managed infection, wound healing problems, and bone healing problems, there were no differences across the groups.[58]

Although conflicting evidence exists regarding the timing of wound closure, most orthopedic surgeons continue to abide by the original work of Gustilo and Anderson. "If there is the slightest doubt in the surgeon's mind as to whether there has been an adequate debridement of the wound after an open fracture, the wound should not be closed regardless of the type of open fracture."[2]

SUMMARY

Open fractures pose an increased risk of infection and require prompt attention and treatment. It is likely that multiple factors including fracture severity, adequacy of debridement, time to initial treatment, and antibiotic administration, among other variables, all contribute to the likelihood of infection and complicate isolating an optimal time to debridement. There is conflicting and insufficient evidence to suggest that debridement of all open fractures in accordance with the historical 6-hour reduces the risk of infection. However, unnecessarily delaying management of open fractures has not been shown to be appropriate. It is consistent with the information in this review to recommend debridement be performed once the patient is adequately resuscitated and stable for surgery with trained staff available. Early administration of appropriate antibiotics has been shown to be a critical factor in reducing and treating the open fracture, and delays in receipt of antibiotics should be considered in managing infection risk. The process of definitive fixation and wound coverage begins with the initial debridement, focusing on bony stability and infection prevention, while also taking into account patient comorbidities and overall nutrition and health status. The combined experience of the orthopedic and plastic surgeon in assessing the soft tissue and bony injury will improve patient care and favor earlier reconstruction, when appropriate. Until such a time when quality studies provide better evidence of the effect of delays in treatment on infection, surgeons should maintain a sense of urgency, but perhaps not emergency, in surgical debridement of open fractures.

REFERENCES

1. Olson SA. Open fractures of the tibial shaft. Current treatment. J Bone Joint Surg Am 1996;78: 1428–37.
2. Gustilo RB, Anderson JT. Prevention of infection in the treatment of one thousand and twenty-five open fractures of long bones: retrospective and prospective analyses. J Bone Joint Surg Am 1976; 58A:453–8.
3. Shtarker H, David R, Stolero J, et al. Treatment of open tibial fractures with primary suture and Ilizarov fixation. Clin Orthop Relat Res 1997;335: 268–74.
4. Russell GG, Henderson R, Arnett G. Primary or delayed closure for open tibial fractures. J Bone Joint Surg Am 1990;72B:125–8.
5. Reuss BL, Cole JD. Effect of delayed treatment on open tibial shaft fractures. Am J Orthop (Belle Mead NJ) 2007;36:215–20.
6. Khatod M, Botte MJ, Hoyt DB, et al. Outcomes in open tibia fractures: relationship between delay in treatment and infection. J Trauma 2003;55:949–54.
7. Hertel R, Lambert SM, Muller S, et al. On the timing of soft-tissue reconstruction for open fractures of the lower leg. Arch Orthop Trauma Surg 1999; 119:7–12.
8. Harley BJ, Beaupre LA, Jones CA, et al. The effect of time to definitive treatment on the rate of nonunion and infection in open fractures. J Orthop Trauma 2002;16:484–90.
9. Crowley DJ, Kanakaris NK, Giannoudis PV. Debridement and wound closure of open fractures: the impact of the time factor on infection rates. Injury 2007;38:879–89.
10. Cole J, Ansel L, Scwartzberg R. A sequential protocol for the management of severe open tibia fractures. Clin Orthop Relat Res 1995;315:84–103.
11. Bednar DA, Parikh J. Effect of time delay from injury to primary management on the incidence of deep infection after open fractures of the lower extremities caused by blunt trauma in adults. J Orthop Trauma 1993;7:532–5.
12. Yang EC, Eisler J. Treatment of isolated type I open fractures: is emergent operative debridement necessary? Clin Orthop Relat Res 2003;410:289–94.
13. Skaggs DL, Friend L, Alman B, et al. The effect of surgical delay on acute infection following 554 open fractures in children. J Bone Joint Surg Am 2005;87:8–12.
14. van den Baar MT, van der Palen J, Vroon MI, et al. Is time to closure a factor in the occurrence of infection in traumatic wounds? A prospective cohort study in a Dutch level 1 trauma centre. Emerg Med J 2010;27:540–3.
15. Schenker ML, Yannascoli S, Baldwin KD, et al. Does timing to operative debridement affect infectious

complications in open long-bone fractures? A systematic review. J Bone Joint Surg Am 2012;94: 1057–64.

16. Friedrich PL. Die aseptische Versorgung frischer Wunden, unter Mittheilung von Thier-Versuchen uber die Auskeimungszeit von Infectionserregern in frischen Wunden. Langenbecks Archiv fur Klinsche Chirugie 1898;288–310.

17. Trueta J. Closed treatment of war fractures. Lancet 1939;1:1452–5.

18. DeLong WG, Born CT, Wei SY, et al. Aggressive treatment of 119 open fracture wounds. J Trauma 1999;46:1049–54.

19. Sungaran J, Harris I, Mourad M. The effect of time to theatre on infection rate for open tibia fractures. ANZ J Surg 2007;77:886–8.

20. Srour M, Inaba K, Okoye O, et al. Prospective evaluation of treatment of open fractures: effect of time to irrigation and debridement. JAMA Surg 2015; 150:332–6.

21. Pollak AN. Timing of débridement of open fractures. J Am Acad Orthop Surg 2006;14:48–51.

22. Giannoudis PV, Papakostidis C, Roberts C. A review of the management of open fractures of the tibia and femur. J Bone Joint Surg Br 2006;88:281–9.

23. Melvin JS, Dombroski DG, Torbert JT, et al. Open tibial shaft fractures: I. Evaluation and initial wound management. J Am Acad Orthop Surg 2010;18:10–9.

24. Court-Brown CM, Rimmer S, Prakash U, et al. The epidemiology of open long bone fractures. Injury 1998;29:529–34.

25. Court-Brown CM, Bulger KE, Clement ND, et al. The epidemiology of open fractures in adults. A 15-year review. Injury 2012;43:891–7.

26. Gustilo RB, Mendoza RM, Williams DN. Problems in the management of type III (severe) open fractures: a new classification of type III open fractures. J Trauma 1984;24:742–6.

27. Tripuraneni K, Ganga S, Quinn R, et al. The effect of time delay to surgical debridement of open tibia shaft fractures on infection rate. Orthopedics 2008;31(12):174–9.

28. Al-Arabi YB, Nader M, Hamidian-Jahromi AR, et al. The effect of the timing of antibiotics and surgical treatment on infection rates in open long-bone fractures: a 9-year prospective study from a district general hospital. Injury 2007;38:900–5.

29. Templeman DC, Gulli B, Tsukayama DT, et al. Update on the management of open fractures of the tibial shaft. Clin Orthop Relat Res 1998;350:18–25.

30. Hannigan GD, Hodkinson BP, McGinnis K, et al. Culture-independent pilot study of microbiota colonizing open fractures and association with severity, mechanism, location, and complication from presentation to early outpatient follow-up. J Orthop Res 2014;32:597–605.

31. Patzakis MJ, Harvey JP, Ivier D. The role of antibiotics in the management of open fractures. J Bone Joint Surg Am 1974;56:532–41.

32. Patzakis MJ, Wilkins J. Factors influencing infection rate in open fracture wounds. Clin Orthop Relat Res 1989;243:36–40.

33. Kim PH, Leopold SS. Gustilo-Anderson classification. Clin Orthop Relat Res 2012;470:32704.

34. Cross WW, Swiontkowski MF. Treatment principles in the management of open fractures. Indian J Orthop 2008;42:377–86.

35. Brumback RJ, Jones AL. Interobserver agreement in the classification of open fractures of the tibia: the results of a survey of two hundred and forty-five orthopaedic surgeons. J Bone Joint Surg Am 1994;76:1162–6.

36. Orthopaedic Trauma Association: Open Fracture Study Group. A new classification scheme for open fractures. J Orthop Trauma 2010;24:457–64.

37. Sirkin M, Liporace F, Behrens FF. Fractures with soft tissue injuries. In: Browner BD, Jupiter JB, Levine AM, et al, editors. Skeletal trauma: basic science, management, and reconstruction. 3rd edition. Philadelphia: Saunders; 2003. p. 367–96.

38. Hoff WS, Bonadies JA, Cachecho R, et al. East practice management guidelines work group: update to practice management guidelines for prophylactic antibiotic use in open fractures. J Trauma 2011;70:751–4.

39. Mundhi R, Chaudhry H, Niroopan G, et al. Open tibial fractures: updated guidelines for management. JBJS Rev 2015;3:e1.

40. Lack WD, Karunakar MA, Angerame MR, et al. Type III open tibia fractures: immediate antibiotic prophylaxis minimizes infection. J Orthop Trauma 2015;29:1–6.

41. Craig J, Fuchs T, Jenks M, et al. Systematic review and meta-analysis of the additional benefit of local prophylactic antibiotic therapy for infection rates in open tibia fractures treated with intramedullary nailing. Int Orthop 2014;38:1025–30.

42. Osterman PA, Henry SL, Seligson D. The role of local antibiotic therapy in the management of compound fractures. Clin Orthop Relat Res 1993;295: 102–11.

43. Werner CM, Pierpont Y, Pollak AN. The urgency of surgical debridement in the management of open fractures. J Am Acad Orthop Surg 2008;16:369–75.

44. Fulkerson EW, Egol KA. Timing issues in fracture management: a review of current concepts. Bull NYU Hosp Jt Dis 2009;67:58–67.

45. Kreder HJ, Armstrong P. A review of open tibia fractures in children. J Pediatr Orthop 1995;15: 482–8.

46. Kindsfater K, Jonassen EA. Osteomyelitis in grade II and III open tibia fractures with late debridement. J Orthop Trauma 1995;9:121–7.

47. Jacob E, Erpelding JM, Murphy KP. A retrospective analysis of open fractures sustained by U.S. military personnel during operation just cause. Mil Med 1992;157:552–6.

48. Penn-Barwell JG, Murray CK, Wenke JC. Early antibiotics and debridement independently reduce infection in an open fracture model. J Bone Joint Surg Am 2012;94:107–12.

49. Ashford RU, Mehta JA, Cripps R. Delayed presentation is no barrier to satisfactory outcome in the management of open tibial fractures. Injury 2004; 35:411–6.

50. Dellinger EP, Miller SD, Wertz MJ, et al. Risk of infection after open fracture of the arm or leg. Arch Surg 1988;123:1320–7.

51. Lenarz CJ, Watson JT, Moed BR, et al. Timing of wound closure in open fractures based on cultures obtained after debridement. J Bone Joint Surg Am 2010;92:1921–6.

52. Lee J. Efficacy of cultures in the management of open fractures. Clin Orthop Relat Res 1997;339: 71–5.

53. Gustilo RB. Use of antimicrobial in the management of open fractures. Arch Surg 1979;114:805–8.

54. Weber D, Dulai SK, Bergman J, et al. Time to initial operative treatment following open fracture does not impact development of deep infection: a prospective cohort study of 736 subjects. J Orthop Trauma 2014;28:613–9.

55. Stannard JP, Volgas DA, Stewart R, et al. Negative pressure wound therapy after severe open fractures: a prospective randomized study. J Orthop Trauma 2009;23:552–7.

56. Hohmann E, Tetsworth K, Radziejowski MJ, et al. Comparison of delayed and primary wound closure in the treatment of open tibial fractures. Arch Orthop Trauma Surg 2007;127:131–6.

57. Bhandari M, Adili A, Schemitsch EH. The efficacy of low-pressure lavage with different irrigating solutions to remove adherent bacteria from bone. J Bone Joint Surg Am 2001;83A:412–9.

58. The FLOW Investigators. A trial of wound irrigation in the initial management of open fracture wounds. N Engl J Med 2015;373:2629–41.

59. Petrisor B, Jeray K, Schemitsch EH, et al. Fluid lavage in patients with open fracture wounds (FLOW): an international survey of 984 surgeons. BMC Musculoskelet Disord 2008;9:7.

60. Anglen JO. Comparison of soap and antibiotic solutions for irrigation of lower-limb open fracture wounds. A prospective, randomized study. J Bone Joint Surg Am 2005;87:1415–22.

Heterotopic Ossification in Trauma

William R. Barfield, PhD, Robert E. Holmes, MD, Langdon A. Hartsock, MD*

KEYWORDS

- Heterotopic ossification • Pathophysiology • Classification • Chemical prophylaxis • Radiation
- Surgical debridement • Surgical excision

KEY POINTS

- Formation of heterotopic ossification (HO) is poorly understood but is an area of continued scientific investigation.
- Certain injuries and patient populations seem to have increased risk of HO formation.
- Brooker classification is most commonly used; however, the Hastings and Graham classification may be more useful around the elbow.
- Pharmacologic agents and radiation have been used in HO prophylaxis.
- Surgical excision is an option for established, symptomatic HO.

INTRODUCTION

Heterotopic ossification (HO), simply stated, is bone that forms where it does not belong. HO can form after trauma, burns, head injuries, spinal cord injuries, and surgical procedures, such as total hip arthroplasty. HO is categorized into neurogenic, thermal, and traumatic types. Neurogenic HO occurs after traumatic brain injury or spinal cord injury. HO can form after thermal injury and is correlated with the overall body surface that has been burned.[1] Traumatic HO occurs after blunt, penetrating, or explosive injuries. All forms of HO may have common elements of pathophysiology; however, detailed information about the pathophysiology at the cellular or protein level has not yet been determined for each type. All types of HO need 3 essential components: pluripotential cells, molecular signals to cause the cells to differentiate, and the proper microenvironment to form bone. Most likely all forms of HO occur because of some amount of tissue trauma, some degree of ischemia, and activation of pluripotential mesenchymal cells, perhaps in part caused by bone morphogenetic protein (BMP).[2]

New osteoblasts form bone in the soft tissues, especially around joints. Heterotopic bone can cross anatomic planes between muscle and tissue layers and can impinge on, or even enclose, neurovascular structures. Heterotopic bone may cause pain because of compression of overlying skin and subcutaneous tissue or because of compression of adjacent structures. Severe HO can cause restriction of joint motion. There is often accompanying fibrosis around the affected joint. The loss of motion can lead to gait disturbances and inability to perform common daily activities such as sitting or eating. The hips and elbows are the most commonly involved joints after trauma and HO is often related to surgery to repair intra-articular fractures in these joints.[3,4] HO may be more common in men and African Americans.[5] The 2 most commonly used methods to prevent HO are use of nonsteroidal antiinflammatory drugs (NSAIDs) and radiation. Treatment of established HO can range from observation, to physical therapy, to surgical excision.

PATHOPHYSIOLOGY OF FORMATION OF HETEROTOPIC OSSIFICATION

The pathophysiology and basic science of HO formation is incompletely understood. Following injury, cellular and molecular signaling

Department of Orthopaedics, Medical University of South Carolina, 96 Jonathan Lucas Street-Suite 708, Charleston, SC 29425, USA
* Corresponding author.
E-mail address: hartsock@musc.edu

Orthop Clin N Am 48 (2017) 35–46
http://dx.doi.org/10.1016/j.ocl.2016.08.009
0030-5898/17/© 2016 Elsevier Inc. All rights reserved.

differentiate dormant, mesenchymal precursor cells that develop into osseous and/or endochondral cells.[6] HO formation, regardless of the injury mechanism (soft tissue trauma, head injury, and spinal cord injury) occurs in soft tissue. Damage to the skeletal muscle with some level of hemorrhage is a predisposing factor. An ischemic environment and activation of pluripotential cells leads to the formation of ectopic bone. BMP may play a role in the differentiation of pluripotential cells into osteoblasts. Mesenchymal stem cells increase osteogenic BMP-2 and BMP-4 expression. The cells are also affected by oxygen tension, micronutrient availability, and mechanical stimuli, leading to increased osteogenesis and potential HO formation.[2,7] Forsberg and colleagues[8] showed that combat wound inflammatory markers increased HO risk. Interleukin (IL)-3 and IL-13 generated by T lymphocytes during wound healing are inhibitors of osteoblastic differentiation and both were found to be independently associated with increased HO risk. Thirteen genes were upregulated in patients who eventually developed HO.[8] Evans and colleagues[9] sought to characterize the expression of osteogenesis-related gene transcription in 54 high-energy penetrating traumatic extremity combat wounds. Their data supported the theory that ectopic bone formation is initiated shortly following the traumatic extremity insult. HO development was noted to occur in tissue environments with a protracted increased inflammatory process, which likely accounts for higher levels of messenger RNA transcription seen at final debridement.[9] Rossier and colleagues,[10] in the 1970s, noted that histologically HO starts shortly after trauma with the proliferation of spindle cells within the first 7 days. During the second week, immature cartilage and woven bone are seen, with trabecular bone forming 2 to 5 weeks following the initial insult. By 6 weeks, undifferentiated central foci form, with mature lamellar bone being located peripherally. Amorphous calcium phosphate is gradually converted to hydroxyapatite crystals and, by 6 months, spicules of bone can be seen within the muscle planes.[10]

Davis and colleagues[6] examined HO risk through muscle biopsies of soldiers injured by high-energy gunshots and blasts compared with patients who had undergone a hamstring tendon autograft. Patients with gunshot and blast injuries showed significantly increased levels of connective tissue progenitor cells per gram of tissue committed to osteogenic differentiation compared with the hamstring autograft group.

Twenty-five percent of US military personnel who sustain extremity amputations as a result of combat have bilateral amputations. Bilateral amputees (BLAs) were compared with a control group that also sustained blast injuries. The BLA group showed increases in the levels of systemic and local wound proinflammatory cytokines, including IL-6 (serum), tumor necrosis factor alpha (exudate), and IL-1 (exudate). The BLA group also had higher rates of wound dehiscence and HO.[11]

EVALUATION OF PATIENTS WITH HETEROTOPIC OSSIFICATION

Patients with HO typically complain of limited range of motion of the affected joint as well as pain and limited function. In the upper extremity this may cause restricted range of motion in the elbow leading to difficulties with activities of daily living, such as eating and grooming. In the hips HO may result in pain, gait disturbance, limp, and difficulty sitting or using the toilet. A careful history should be conducted to evaluate for past medical history, trauma, head injury, spinal cord injury, and any previous surgery. Examine the patient for range of motion, strength, and any neurovascular abnormalities. The imaging work-up starts with plain radiographs, which are easy to obtain and inexpensive. On the radiograph the extent of the HO can be seen. A computed tomography (CT) scan with three-dimensional reconstruction gives detailed visualization of HO. HO often crosses anatomic fascial planes and can be very close to important neurovascular structures. In patients after open reduction and internal fixation (ORIF) of acetabular fracture, HO is almost always in the location of the previous surgery. Because the Kocher-Langenbeck approach is the most commonly used, HO usually involves the hip abductors and short external rotators. Typically, the sciatic nerve cannot be definitively visualized by CT, but HO is often near the nerve and can occasionally encase the nerve. Other studies, such as bone scans and single-photon emission CT scans, can help with understanding the metabolic activity of the bone, but are not useful in terms of planning a surgical excision because these studies lack the detailed resolution of a CT scan.

HETEROTOPIC OSSIFICATION IN THE UPPER EXTREMITY

HO has been described in the upper extremity, although its incidence is much less common than in other areas of the body. HO of the shoulder has been described following anterior acromioplasty, with an incidence reported from 3% to 30%.[12–15]

HO incidence after proximal humerus fractures has not been well described in the literature, although it is a known complication.[16] HO formation of the upper extremity most commonly occurs in the elbow, frequently after the so-called terrible triad injuries and after comminuted distal humerus fractures or fracture dislocations (Figs. 1 and 2). Most commonly, HO occurs in the posterolateral aspect of the elbow, extending from the lateral humeral condyle to the posterolateral olecranon. Ectopic bone can fill the olecranon fossa, which leads to deficits in terminal extension. HO may also occur at the coronoid, especially after terrible triad injuries. This condition may inhibit flexion and lead to coronoid impingement (Figs. 3 and 4). Morrey and colleagues[17] reported that a 100° arc of motion was necessary for 90% of functional activities about the elbow. In many cases, HO can severely limit this motion and may lead to significant functional deficits, including issues with performance of activities of daily living. HO around the elbow can be classified according to the Hastings and Graham classification system (Table 1). Occasionally HO can be seen on the anterior aspect of the elbow, and can extend from the anterior humerus to the radius and the ulna to the level of the bicipital tuberosity. This condition may lead to a radioulnar synostosis or median or radial nerve palsy.[18,19]

The magnitude of local tissue trauma sustained in an injury seems to predispose the development of HO.[20] In general, HO likelihood increases with the severity of injury. Likewise, the degree of surgery also correlates with the likelihood of HO formation. Several studies have shown a link between operative time, extent of surgical dissection, and number of surgeries as predisposing factors for HO formation. In addition, many investigators theorize that dissemination of bone dust or debris, as well as hematoma formation, can predispose to HO formation.[20,21]

HETEROTOPIC OSSIFICATION IN THE LOWER EXTREMITY

Pain can occur from prominence of the HO under the skin and subcutaneous tissue. Commonly this is on the lateral side of the hip. HO can form after a variety of surgical procedures around the hip, including hip arthroplasty, hip arthroscopy, fixation of acetabular fractures, or proximal femur fractures, as well as intramedullary nailing of femur fractures (Figs. 5 and 6). Typically bone forms in the abductor muscles adjacent to the entry site of the intramedullary nail in the proximal femur. This condition can cause localized pain directly at the site of the HO.

Internal fixation of acetabular fractures can lead to the formation of HO. The Kocher-Langenbeck approach and the extended iliofemoral approach are most often implicated in the formation of HO after ORIF of acetabular fractures,[8] but HO formation is highly variable. In most cases there is no HO or very small amounts correlating with Brooker stage I (Table 2). Predisposing factors may exist for patients who get Brooker stage III or IV HO after fixation of an acetabular fracture. Some investigators have

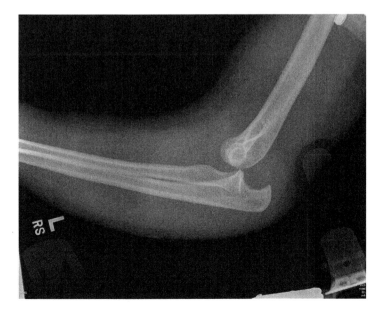

Fig. 1. Lateral view of unstable elbow dislocation.

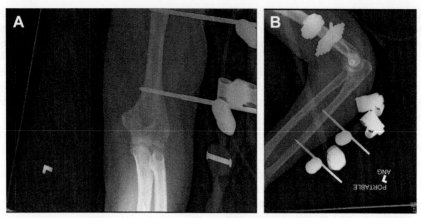

Fig. 2. (A) Anteroposterior (AP) and (B) lateral views of unstable elbow in a hinged external fixator.

implicated surgical approach, sex, race, as well as associated injuries such as a closed head injury.[8]

Pain may occur when the patient tries to sleep or lie on the affected hip. Pain may also occur from compression of neurovascular structures around the hip. Compression of the sciatic nerve at the level of the hip by HO can lead to neuropathic pain, numbness, or weakness in the leg.[22]

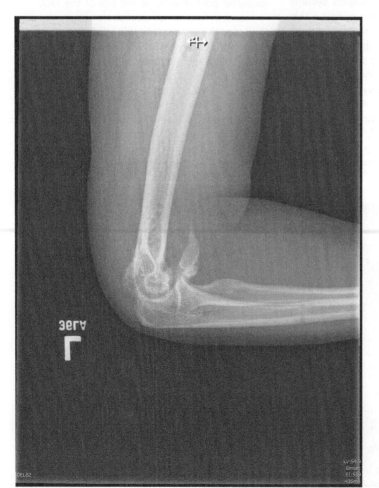

Fig. 3. Lateral view of same elbow, which now has HO that limits motion.

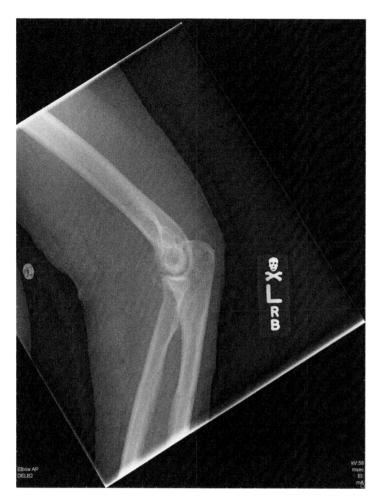

Fig. 4. Lateral view of same elbow after HO excision.

Table 1
The Hastings and Graham classification of HO around the elbow

Hastings and Graham HO Classification	Extent of HO
Ectopic bone without functional limitation	I
Functional limitation of F/E	IIA
Functional limitation of P/S	IIB
Functional limitation of F/E and P/S	IIC
Bony ankylosis completely restricts F/E	IIIA
Bony ankylosis completely restricts P/S	IIIB
Bony ankylosis completely restricts F/E and P/S	IIIC

Abbreviations: F/E, flexion/extension; P/S, pronation/supination.

HETEROTOPIC OSSIFICATION AROUND THE HIP

Most HO around the hip is minor to moderate (Brooker grades I–II). This amount of HO does not usually significantly impede range of motion around the hip. Most commonly this occurs after hip replacement surgery. In trauma, the most common fracture related to the development of HO is an acetabular fracture. A report by Griffin and colleagues[20] noted that the overall incidence of HO after ORIF of acetabular fractures through a posterior approach was 47%. Twenty-six percent of the patients had Brooker grades I or II, 13% had Brooker grade III, and 8% had Brooker grade IV. Overall, 15% of patients became symptomatic and 3.3% underwent HO excision.[20] Griffin and colleagues[20] found a 12% incidence of Brooker II or IV HO after ORIF of acetabular fractures via a posterior (Kocher-Langenbeck) approach. Patients with Brooker grade III or IV HO may have near-complete or complete ankylosis of the joint

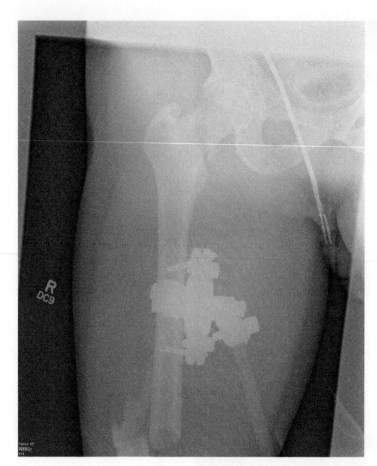

Fig. 5. AP view of femoral neck fracture caused by high-energy trauma.

caused by bone completely bridging from one side of the joint to the other (see Fig. 6). The stiffness is caused by the block of motion from bone formation around the joint. In addition, there is also periarticular fibrosis, which contributes to the joint stiffness.

HO limits the patient's ability to work, play, and perform activities of daily living, such as sitting, dressing, bathing, or using the toilet. The loss of motion can lead to inability to use the joint and the joint can essentially be fused in a nonfunctional position.

Most reports do not indicate a difference in development of HO by race, gender, or age. However, a recent report on patients undergoing excision of HO around the hip found a higher incidence of severe HO requiring resection in African American men.[5]

HETEROTOPIC OSSIFICATION IN COMBAT INJURIES

HO has been reported in United States military records as far back as the Civil War. However, recent conflicts have been responsible for extremely high rates of HO formation in military injured populations. In one study, 63% of military casualties developed radiographically apparent HO. Improved medical technology and military defense equipment has increased the likelihood of patients surviving injuries that may have proven fatal in years past. One recent study reported that 90% of soldiers who become combat casualties survive their injuries. Advances in advance trauma life support protocols have greatly diminished mortality from extremity trauma in both military and civilian populations. In addition, field tourniquet use, improved surgical techniques, and resuscitative abilities, as well as highly advanced personal protective gear, make survival more likely.

In a recent study of military populations involved in the conflicts of Iraq and Afghanistan, several factors correlated with the risk of developing HO. These factors included blast injury, amputation through the zone of injury, and traumatic brain injury.

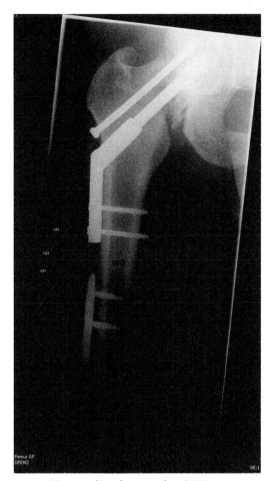

Fig. 6. AP view of hip fracture after ORIF.

BLAST INJURIES IN WAR

Many investigators theorize that HO formation is a result of an unregulated inflammatory response after significant trauma. Several studies have shown that blast injuries, especially traumatic amputations, have a higher rate of HO formation than penetrating injuries. Several

Table 2
The Brooker classification of HO around the hip

Brooker HO Classification	Stage
No heterotopic bone	0
Islands of bone in soft tissue	1
Bone spurs with 1 cm between bones	2
Bone spurs with <1 cm between bones	3
Bony ankylosis	4

factors may contribute to the phenomenon. First, patients who have blast injuries are much more likely to have a concomitant traumatic brain injury, or other injury to the central nervous system, which has been shown to lead to HO formation. Second, blast injuries create a massive inflammatory response in local tissues. This major bone and soft tissue trauma results in dysregulation of the normal healing response, leading to ectopic bone formation. Both the magnitude of the blast trauma and the resulting treatment can contribute to the formation of HO.[6,8] When amputation must be performed, many surgeons perform the amputation through the zone of injury in order to conserve as much limb as possible. The nature of a blast means that the zone of injury sustained is larger than in other types of injuries. Although limb conservation is a worthy goal, HO may form in the residual stump (Fig. 7), causing chronic pain and leading to loss of function, including difficulty with the use of prosthetics devices.[23]

PROPHYLACTIC MODALITIES
Pharmacologic
NSAIDs reduce HO risk by limiting osteogenic differentiation of progenitor cells.[18] Indomethacin, a nonselective cyclooxygenase (COX) 1

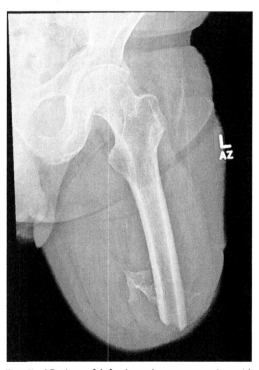

Fig. 7. AP view of left above-knee amputation with HO at distal end of stump causing difficulty with wearing prosthesis.

and COX 2 inhibitor, is commonly dosed at 75 mg twice per day, although the timing and magnitude of dosing specifics have yet to be completely studied.[19] One study supports the use of no indomethacin following acetabular fracture. Griffin and colleagues[20] found that, among 120 patients treated for acetabular fractures with the Kocher-Langenbeck approach, there were no differences between the incidence of moderate (Brooker class III) and severe HO (Brooker class IV) when indomethacin and placebo groups from a historical study were compared. Based on these findings indomethacin use was discontinued. HO risk after hip resurfacing is higher than for patients who have a total hip arthroplasty. Aspirin, a nonselective NSAID, reduces the severity and incidence of HO risk following hip resurfacing to levels similar to that seen for patients with total hip arthroplasty.[24] The use of NSAIDs to reduce HO risk must be balanced against the risk for long bone and acetabular nonunion.[21,25]

Bisphosphonates induce osteoclast apoptosis and reduce bony calcification, but their use as prophylactic agents in HO reduction is controversial, with some studies supporting use and others finding this therapy ineffective.[2]

A comprehensive, moderate-quality meta-analysis from 2015 found that NSAIDs reduce the incidence of HO following total hip arthroplasty, but increase the risk of gastrointestinal side effects. Selective NSAIDs did not differ from nonselective NSAIDs in prevention of HO, but selective NSAIDs produced fewer side effects. Despite the benefits of selective NSAIDs for HO prophylaxis, longer follow-up is needed to balance the risk/benefit ratio.[26]

Radiation

Radiotherapy (RT) has been shown to provide effective HO prophylaxis and is commonly administered from 1 to 5 days postoperatively.[12] Postoperative dosing is much more common than preoperative dosing with acetabular fractures because patients are more comfortable and confident transferring from the bed to the scanner after stabilization of the fracture.[12] One recent study compared the effectiveness of preoperative with postoperative radiation for HO prophylaxis in the treatment of acetabular fractures. No statistical differences in HO frequency or severity were noted in their study, although because of low numbers the investigation was likely underpowered to reveal a difference.[27] Commonly, a single 8-Gy dose is administered at energies between 6 and 15 MV, with higher energies

needed for larger patients.[12] Historically, RT HO prophylaxis was administered in smaller doses of 2 Gy over 5 to 10 fractions for a total of 10 to 20 Gy,[10,11] but recent studies have shown the treatment efficacy of single-fraction doses of 7 Gy or more.[13,15] RT has associated malignancy risk and there have been 2 case reports of radiation-induced sarcoma associated with RT after HO prophylaxis: 1 sarcoma developing 18 years after two 7-Gy doses, and another sarcoma 11 years after a single 7-Gy dose.[16,28] Although this information is important, without knowing the denominator and numbers of patients who had successful HO treatment without malignancy, estimates of incidence are not possible. Death risk from a fatal radiation-induced malignancy is highly variable, from 1 in 1000 to 1 in 10,000; however, credible midranges are based on age and are generally between 1 in 2000 for younger patients and 1 in 6000 for older patients. Indomethacin prophylaxis has been shown to be less effective in HO prophylaxis, with higher death risk from complications of 1 in 900.[12] Side effects of radiation beyond the risk of malignancy include increased risk of soft tissue contracture, delayed wound healing, nonunion, and compromised bony ingrowth with press-fit hip prostheses. The efficacy of radiation to reduce HO in joints other than the hip has not been adequately studied.[29]

Surgical Debridement of Damaged Muscle

There are no reports of a surgical topical or injectable agent to prevent formation of HO. Careful surgical technique, excision of damaged muscle, and avoidance of postoperative hematoma are important. Rath and colleagues[30] reported on the excision of necrotic gluteus minimus muscle at the conclusion of ORIF of acetabular fracture repair surgery. HO occurred in 12 of 29 patients, but Brooker grade II or IV HO occurred in only 3 patients.

TREATMENT OF ESTABLISHED HETEROTOPIC OSSIFICATION

Minor Heterotopic Ossification

In most patients HO is minor and does not cause a significant loss of motion or pain. Sometimes HO is revealed as an incidental finding on a routine radiograph taken to evaluate another symptom related to the joint in question. Most of these small areas of HO do not significantly affect joint range of motion or activities of daily living. These small islands of HO can be observed and no specific intervention is required. Occasionally, a small area of HO forms adjacent to

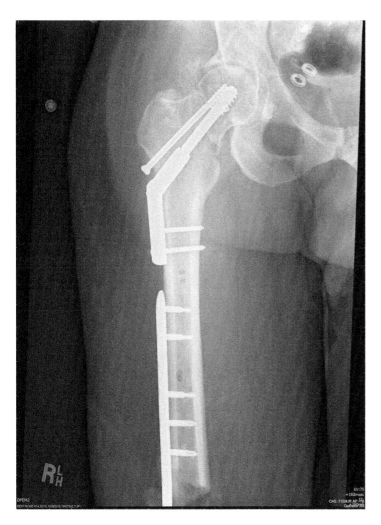

Fig. 8. AP view of left hip with grade IV HO causing complete ankyloses of hip. The HO bridges from the ilium to the lateral neck of the femur.

the subcutaneous aspect of a bone such as the lateral margin of the greater trochanter. If this area causes chronic pain surgery may be indicated to remove the painful HO.

Major Heterotopic Ossification

Major HO results in stiffness and pain, and in some cases can impede joint motion. The HO can be excised, but this can be technically

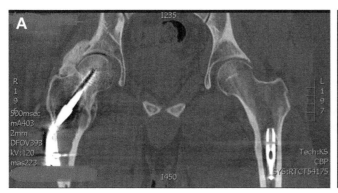
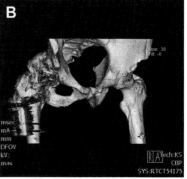

Fig. 9. (A) Coronal CT and (B) three-dimensional reconstruction of pelvis showing right hip HO.

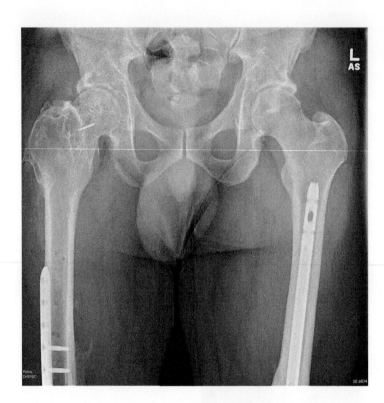

Fig. 10. AP view of hip after excision of HO and removal of hardware.

difficult (**Figs. 8** and **9**). The surgery can result in significant blood loss and requires preoperative crossmatching to make sure blood is available. Adjacent neurovascular structures are at risk because of substantial altered anatomy. Patients usually obtain a greater range of motion after surgery and intensive postoperative rehabilitation[31] (see **Fig. 7**).

HO bone forms in and across typical tissue planes, which can result in altered and confusing tissue anatomy. Nerves and vessels can be displaced or encased in the HO tissue. Surgical removal is possible, but can be hazardous to adjacent neurovascular structures, which are difficult to visualize in and around the heterotopic bone. The joint can be damaged if there is not a clear demarcation between HO and natural bone. During surgery, HO bone is isolated from adjacent soft tissues and excised (see **Fig. 8**). The amount of bone, especially around the hip, can vary and in some cases can be large. After excision the resultant dead space needs to be reduced and postoperative hematomas should be avoided (see **Fig. 9**). Usually these patients get postoperative radiation to prevent recurrence. Patients should start on immediate range-of-motion therapy to prevent recurrence of contracture (**Fig. 10**).

SUMMARY

Better understanding of the biology of HO formation will lead to treatment and prevention modalities that can be directed specifically at the cellular level. Early identification of HO precursor cells and target genes may provide prognostic value that guides individualized prophylactic treatment of patients at highest risk of development of HO. Better understanding of molecular signaling and proteomics variability will allow surgeons to individualize preemptive treatment to suppress inflammation and formation of HO.

Primary prevention of HO is currently performed by using prophylactic doses of nonsteroidal antiinflammatory medications or a single dose of radiation to the affected area in the immediate postoperative period, usually within 72 hours. Careful surgical technique to avoid muscle damage is important. Damaged muscle should be debrided as a prophylactic measure to prevent formation of HO around the joint. In addition, hemostasis and avoidance of a postoperative hematoma may decrease the chance of formation of HO.

REFERENCES

1. Cartotto R, Cicuto BJ, Kiwanuka HN, et al. Common postburn deformities and their

management. Surg Clin North Am 2014;94(4): 817–37.

2. Ranganathan K, Loder S, Agarwal S, et al. Heterotopic ossification: basic-science principles and clinical correlates. J Bone Joint Surg Am 2015;97:1101–11.

3. Ozturk BY, Kelly BT. Heterotopic ossification in portal sites following hip arthroscopy. Arch Orthop Trauma Surg 2014;133(7):979–84.

4. Hong CC, Nashi N, Hey HW, et al. Clinically relevant heterotopic ossification after elbow fracture surgery: a risk factors study. Orthop Traumatol Surg Res 2015;101(2):209–13.

5. Slone HS, Walton ZJ, Daly CA, et al. The impact of race on the development of severe heterotopic ossification following acetabular fracture surgery. Injury 2015;46(6):1069–73.

6. Davis TA, O'Brien FP, Anam K, et al. Heterotopic ossification in complex orthopaedic combat wounds. J Bone Joint Surg Am 2011;93:1122–31.

7. Salisbury E, Rodenberg E, Sonnet C, et al. Sensory nerve induced inflammation contributes to heterotopic ossification. J Cell Biochem 2011;112(10): 2748–58.

8. Forsberg JA, Potter BK, Polfer EM, et al. Do inflammatory markers portend heterotopic ossification and wound failure in combat wounds. Clin Orthop Relat Res 2014;472:2845–54.

9. Evans KN, Potter BK, Brown TS, et al. Osteogenic gene expression correlates with development of heterotopic ossification in war wounds. Clin Orthop Relat Res 2014;472:396–404.

10. Rossier AB, Bussat P, Infante F, et al. Current facts of para-osteo-arthropathy (POA). Paraplegia 1973; 11(1):38–78.

11. Lisboa FA, Forsberg JA, Brown TS, et al. Bilateral lower-extremity amputation wounds are associated with distinct local and systemic cytokine response. Surgery 2013;154(2):281–90.

12. Burnet NG, Nasr P, Vip G, et al. Prophylactic radiotherapy against heterotopic ossification following internal fixation of acetabular fractures: a comparative estimate of risk. Br J Radiol 2014;87:1042–50.

13. Sylvester JE, Greenberg P, Selch MT, et al. The use of postoperative irradiation for the prevention of heterotopic bone formation after total hip replacement. Int J Radiat Oncol Biol Phys 1988;14:471–6.

14. Lo TC, Healy WL, Covall DJ, et al. Heterotopic bone formation after hip surgery: prevention with single-dose postoperative hip irradiation. Radiology 1988;168:851–4.

15. Mourad WF, Packianathan S, Shourbaji RA, et al. A prolonged time interval between trauma and prophylactic radiation therapy significantly increases the risk of heterotopic ossification. Int J Radiat Oncol Biol Phys 2012;82:339–44.

16. Mourad WF, Packianathan S, Shourbaji RA, et al. Radiation-induced sarcoma following radiation prophylaxis of heterotopic ossification. Pract Radiat Oncol 2012;2:151–4.

17. Morrey BF, Askew LJ, Chao EY. A biomechanical study of normal functional elbow motion. J Bone Joint Surg Am 1981;63(6):872–7.

18. Chang JK, Li CJ, Liao HJ, et al. Anti-inflammatory drugs suppress proliferation and induce apoptosis through altering expressions of cell cycle regulators and pro-apoptotic factors in cultured human osteoblasts. Toxicologist 2009;258:148–56.

19. LeDuff MJ, Takamura KB, Amstutz HC. Incidence of heterotopic ossification and effects of various prophylactic methods after hip resurfacing. Bull NYU Hosp Jt Dis 2011;69:S36–41.

20. Griffin SM, Sims SH, Karunakar MA, et al. Heterotopic ossification rates after acetabular fracture surgery are unchanged without indomethacin prophylaxis. Clin Orthop Relat Res 2013;471:2776–82.

21. Sagi HC, Jordan CJ, Barei DP, et al. Indomethacin prophylaxis for heterotopic ossification after acetabular fracture surgery increases the risk for nonunion of the posterior wall. J Orthop Trauma 2014;28(7):377–83.

22. Polfer EM, Forsberg JA, Fleming ME, et al. Neurovascular entrapment due to combat-related heterotopic ossification in the lower extremity. J Bone Joint Surg Am 2013;95(24):e195(1-6).

23. Brown KV, Dharm-Datta S, Potter BK, et al. Comparison of development of heterotopic ossification in injured US and UK armed services personnel with combat-related amputations: preliminary findings and hypotheses regarding causality. J Trauma 2010;69:S116–22.

24. Nunley RM, Zhu J, Clohisy JC, et al. Aspirin decreases heterotopic ossification after hip resurfacing. Clin Orthop Relat Res 2011;469:1614–20.

25. Pountos I, Georgeuli T, Calori GM, et al. Do nonsteroidal anti-inflammatory drugs affect bone healing? A critical analysis. ScientificWorldJournal 2012;2012:606404.

26. Kan SL, Yang B, Ning GZ, et al. Nonsteroidal anti-inflammatory drugs as prophylaxis for heterotopic ossification after total hip arthroplasty. Medicine (Baltimore) 2015;94(18):e828.

27. Archdeacon MT, d'Heurle A, Nemeth N, et al. Is preoperative radiation therapy as effective as postoperative radiation therapy for heterotopic ossification prevention in acetabular fractures? Clin Orthop Relat Res 2014;472:3389–94.

28. Hamid N, Ashraf N, Bosse MJ, et al. Radiation therapy for heterotopic ossification prophylaxis acutely after elbow trauma: a prospective randomized study. J Bone Joint Surg Am 2010;92(11):2032–8.

29. Farris MK, Chowdhry VK, Lemke S, et al. Osteosarcoma following single fraction radiation prophylaxis for heterotopic ossification. Radiat Oncol 2012;7:140–3.

30. Rath EM, Russell GV Jr, Washington WJ, et al. Gluteus minimus necrotic muscle debridement diminishes heterotopic ossification after acetabular fracture fixation. Injury 2002;33(9):751–6.

31. Wu XB, Yang MH, Zhu SW, et al. Surgical resection of severe heterotopic ossification after open reduction and internal fixation of acetabular fractures: a case series of 18 patients. Injury 2014;45(10):1604–10.

Pediatrics

Clavicle Shaft Fractures in Adolescents

Scott Yang, MD[a], Lindsay Andras, MD[b],*

KEYWORDS

- Adolescent clavicle fractures • Clavicle shaft fractures • Clavicle malunion
- Operative clavicle fracture treatment • Nonoperative clavicle fracture treatment

KEY POINTS

- The optimal treatment of displaced adolescent clavicle fractures remains controversial.
- Nonunions of adolescent clavicle fractures are extremely rare, and treatment generally focuses on prevention of symptomatic malunion.
- Malunions in adolescent clavicle fractures may not result in major deficits as in adults; however, high level evidence is lacking to support this conclusion.

INTRODUCTION

Clavicle shaft fractures are among the most common fractures of the upper extremity in adolescents. The incidence of clavicle shaft fractures in the pediatric population is 15% among all upper extremity injuries.[1] Traditionally, clavicle shaft fractures in children and adolescents have been managed nonoperatively, with the exception of open or impending open fractures and fractures associated with floating shoulders or with neurovascular compromise. Most clavicle fractures occur in the shaft along the middle third; this article focuses specifically on clavicle shaft fractures. The optimal treatment of clavicle shaft fractures for older children and adolescents is a topic of major controversy because the literature has shifted more in favor of surgical treatment of displaced clavicle fractures in adults, although whether the research on outcomes in adults is applicable to this younger population remains debatable.

ANATOMY

The clavicle is an S-shaped bone when viewed from the axial plane and is a key structure to the shoulder girdle. It has 2 articulations: medially at the sternoclavicular joint and laterally at the acromioclavicular joint. The joint capsules provide stability in both craniocaudal and anteroposterior planes while allowing for rotation occurring with the arc of motion of the shoulder. The clavicle is a key structure of the shoulder suspensory complex, providing ligamentous attachments to the scapula via the conoid and trapezoid coracoclavicular ligaments. In children and younger adolescents, these ligaments attach to a thick periosteal sleeve. Six muscles attach to the clavicle, with the sternocleidomastoid, sternohyoid, and pectoralis major attaching medially; the subclavius muscle attaching along the midportion; and the deltoid and trapezius attaching laterally. Understanding the relative muscular attachments allows for appreciation of direction of displacement of fracture fragments (Fig. 1). The clavicle is also an important structure that protects critical neurovascular structures, including the subclavian artery and vein, and the brachial plexus, especially along the middle third of the clavicle.

All authors in this article have no disclosures regarding commercial or financial conflicts of interests, or funding sources for this work.

[a] Orthopaedics and Rehabilitation, Doernbecher Children's Hospital, Oregon Health and Science University, 3181 South West Sam Jackson Park Road, Portland, OR 97239, USA; [b] Children's Orthopaedic Center, Children's Hospital Los Angeles, 4650 Sunset Boulevard, MS#69, Los Angeles, CA 90027, USA
* Corresponding author.
E-mail address: landras@chla.usc.edu

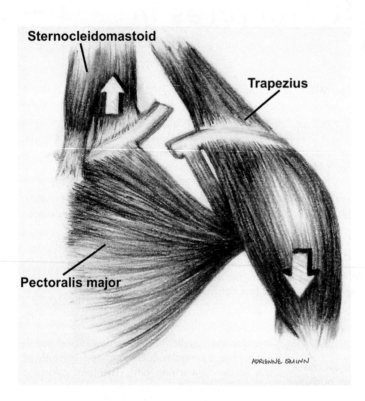

Sternocleidomastoid

Trapezius

Pectoralis major

ADRIENNE QUINN

Fig. 1. Typical displacement of clavicle shaft fracture fragments with the medial fragment pulled cephalad by the sternocleidomastoid and the lateral fragment pulled caudad by the weight of the arm.

GROWTH AND OSSIFICATION OF THE CLAVICLE

The clavicle forms by both endochondral and intramembranous ossification. Its primary central ossification center appears in utero around 5 and one-half weeks, and continues to contribute to most clavicular growth postnatally via intramembranous ossification. The secondary medial and lateral epiphyseal growth centers appear in adolescence and contribute growth at the ends of the clavicle via endochondral ossification. The medial and lateral epiphyseal growth centers fuse around 25 years of age and 19 years of age, respectively.[2] Despite the later appearance and fusion of the epiphyseal growth centers, most clavicular growth occurs earlier in life. McGraw and colleagues[3] demonstrated that 80% of the full length of the clavicle is reached by 9 years in girls, and 12 years in boys. Nonoperative treatment of displaced fractures in children relies heavily on the growth and remodeling potential of the fractured bone. Proponents of surgical treatment of severely displaced clavicle fractures may view the diminished remodeling potential of the clavicle in adolescents as a major factor in proposing treatment plans analogous to those in adults.

MECHANISM OF INJURY AND EVALUATION

The clavicle shaft is most commonly injured by an axial load to the clavicle transmitted through a fall onto the shoulder. Less common mechanisms of fracture include a direct blow to the clavicle or fall onto an outstretched hand. The middle one-third shaft of the clavicle is the most commonly injured location due to its transitional location leading to a stress riser, where the shape of the clavicle transitions from concave to convex, and from tubular to flat. The direction of displacement depends on both the location of the fracture and the initial force causing the injury. Superior displacement of the medial fragment is common due to the pull of the sternocleidomastoid and can lead to tenting of the skin (Fig. 2) or, in rare instances, open injuries when there is severe displacement. The lateral fragment often displaces inferiorly due to the weight of the shoulder and arm. A thorough neurovascular examination of the injured extremity should be performed to due to the proximity of the subclavian vessels and brachial plexus. Severe displacement or comminution of the clavicle fracture should alert the clinician to a high-energy mechanism, and one should be vigilant in looking for potential associated injuries, including pneumothorax, or

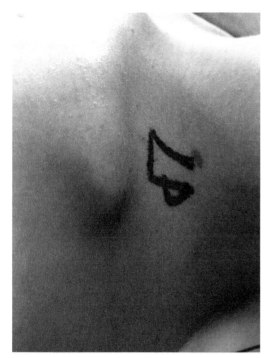

Fig. 2. Skin tenting in a displaced midshaft clavicle fracture.

fractures of the scapula and ribs. Anteroposterior and 30-degree cephalic tilt radiographs (serendipity view) with the patient in an upright position are sufficient to characterize clavicle shaft fractures. In cases of significant comminution, including radiographs of the contralateral side can aid in assessing the amount of shortening.

NONOPERATIVE TREATMENT OPTIONS

Nonoperative treatment generally involves the use of a simple shoulder sling or figure-of-8 brace for approximately 3 to 4 weeks, followed by gradual increase in range of motion. There is an absence of data in the literature supporting that a figure-of-8 brace results in improved outcomes when compared with a shoulder sling, though the figure-of-8 bracing has been associated with more pain and discomfort.[4] Consequently, a shoulder sling has become the preferred nonoperative treatment method. In the adolescent, gradual return to strengthening can be started at 6 weeks, and union should be expected by 12 weeks in most cases. In younger children, fracture healing may be more expeditious.

SURGICAL TREATMENT OPTIONS

Multiple surgical methods have been described for the treatment of clavicle shaft fractures. The most commonly used method is open reduction and internal fixation with an anatomically contoured plate and screw construct. Several studies have also demonstrated excellent results with intramedullary pin fixation for simple fracture patterns.[5–7] Specific advantages of plate fixation include direct visual control of the fracture fragment and biomechanically more rigid fixation. Intramedullary fixation preserves the soft tissue around the fracture sites if a direct open reduction is not used, though complications, including hardware breakage, prominent hardware, skin breakdown near hardware, and pin migration, have been reported.[8] Additionally, in many cases in which surgical stabilization is considered, the fracture patterns are more complex and thus not amenable to intramedullary stabilization. Consequently, this article focuses on open reduction and internal fixation with plate fixation as the primary surgical treatment because this is the method of stabilization in most the recent literature in both adults and adolescents.

SURGICAL TECHNIQUE FOR PLATE AND SCREW FIXATION

For open reduction and internal fixation of clavicle fractures, a superior or anterior plating location can be chosen based on surgeon preference. The patient is positioned in a beach chair or supine position, based on the surgeon's preference. An approximately 7 to 9 cm horizontal skin incision is made centered along the clavicle. The subcutaneous tissue and platysma is dissected and, if visible, the crossing supraclavicular nerves are identified and preserved. Occasionally, a supraclavicular nerve branch is sacrificed to gain adequate exposure for the open reduction and internal fixation, and it is important to counsel the patient about small regions of potential superior chest wall numbness before surgery. The clavipectoral fascia and surrounding muscle is dissected in a clean plane to allow for eventual closure. The bone is exposed with the periosteal elevator. If 1 large comminuted fragment is present, it is reduced to 1 of the major fragments with a small fracture reduction clamp and a lag screw (generally 2.7 mm or 3.5 mm) is inserted to secure the fragment. The surgeon should be careful to preserve some periosteum on the comminuted fragment to help maintain its viability and facilitate fracture healing. Next, the major bone fragments are directly held by fracture reduction clamps and reduced anatomically. If the fracture configuration allows, it is helpful to either place a 1.6 mm k-wire to hold this reduction or place 1 or more lag screws away from the plane of the intended plate to hold the major fragments together. An anatomically contoured plate is assessed for overall fit along the clavicle, with a goal of at least 3 screws on each of the major fracture fragments. Occasionally, the plates require subtle bending to match the clavicle shape and prevent loss of reduction as the screws are affixed to the plate. The screw holes are drilled with care not to plunge in order not to injure lung or underlying neurovascular structures. Screws are sequentially placed on each side of the fracture, the fixation verified fluoroscopically, and routine irrigation and closure is performed. A sling is used postoperatively for comfort for a maximum of 2 weeks and pendulum exercises to the shoulder are allowed. From 2 to 6 weeks range of motion is gradually progressed. From 6 weeks, gradual strengthening of the shoulder can commence and contact sports can be performed once full radiographic union and strength is achieved.

CURRENT CONTROVERSY

Most clavicle fractures in adolescents have been typically treated nonoperatively. The absolute indications for surgery involve open fractures, impending open fractures with skin tenting, and displaced clavicle fractures in the setting of floating shoulders or neurovascular compromise. In the past 10 years, the trends in treating middle third clavicle fractures in adults have changed drastically in favor of open reduction and internal fixation, with an increased annual incidence of clavicle shaft fracture open reduction and internal fixation of 61.5% from 2007 to 2011.[9] This trend was initially spearheaded by a randomized controlled trial by the Canadian Orthopedic Trauma Society, which demonstrated significantly improved functional outcome scores and decreased rates of nonunion with plate fixation of displaced clavicle shaft fractures compared with those of nonoperative treatment (10.8% nonoperative group, 2.98% plate fixation group).[10] In the adult population, clavicle fractures treated nonoperatively have been associated with poorer outcomes and significantly decreased strength and endurance.[10–13] Fractures, particularly with 2 cm of initial shortening, have been shown to be more prone to nonunion.[14] Furthermore, several studies have demonstrated that plate fixation and corrective osteotomy after initial malunion of nonoperatively treated fractures results in significant improvement of subjective and functional outcomes.[12,15] Hence, based on the trifecta of superior strength

and endurance, improved functional outcome scores, and decreased rates of nonunions, surgical treatment of more than 100% displaced or 2 cm shortened clavicle fractures has become the preferred treatment method in adults. Recent treatment trends of clavicle fractures in adolescents have mirrored the enthusiasm of surgical treatment in adults. A national insurance database study demonstrated similar trends in adolescents with significantly increased operative treatment of adolescent clavicle fractures in the 10- to 19-year age group from years 2007 to 2011 (12.5% in 2007 compared with 21.9% in 2011).[16] A major controversy remains about whether the increased trend toward surgical treatment of clavicle shaft fractures in adolescents results in improved clinical outcomes as in adults.

CURRENT TREATMENT OUTCOMES

Although the rate of nonunions in completely displaced adult clavicle fractures has been demonstrated to be up to 15%,[11,17,18] nonunions are exceedingly rare in adolescent clavicle fractures regardless of nonoperative or surgical treatment. Recent studies demonstrate no nonunions of displaced clavicle fractures in adolescents, and only few isolated cases in the literature report on nonunions in children or adolescents.[19–22] Because nonunions rarely occur in adolescents, the main focus of whether surgical treatment offers advantages compared with nonoperative treatment remains in the prevention of malunion and its potential associated functional deficits.

Plate fixation of adolescent clavicle fractures has excellent outcomes with regard to union and functional outcome. Mehlman and colleagues[23] treated 24 children with displaced clavicle fractures via open reduction and plate fixation and reported no nonunions, no infections, and 87% of patients returning to unrestricted sports. Namdari and colleagues[24] demonstrated favorable objective functional QuickDASH (Quick Disabilities of the Arm, Shoulder, and Hand) scores in adolescents of average 12.9 years of age with clavicle fractures treated with plate fixation.

Vander Have and colleagues[25] compared adolescents with clavicle shaft fractures treated with plate fixation versus nonoperative treatment. Although the treatment groups were different with regard to the amount of initial fracture displacement (mean 2.75 cm in plate fixation group, mean 1.25 cm in nonoperative group), the plate fixation group achieved faster time to radiographic union and faster return to normal activities by mean 4 weeks. There were no nonunions in either the nonoperative or plate fixation groups. Although there were no malunions in the plate fixation group, 5 out of 25 subjects (20%) in the nonoperative group developed symptomatic malunion. The subjects who developed symptomatic malunion had mean 2.6 cm of shortening of the fracture site. The most common complication after plate fixation of adolescent clavicle fractures in this study and others is prominent or symptomatic hardware, ranging from 8% to 18%.[25–27] After hardware removal, refracture of the clavicle is a potential complication, as shown in Fig. 3. Rates of infection, neurovascular injury, pneumothorax, or fracture around the plate are not well reported in the literature on adolescents.

More recent studies focus on comparing functional outcomes between nonoperative and surgical treatment of clavicle fractures. Parry and colleagues[26] retrospectively compared 8 adolescents (mean age 14 years, minimum 9 months follow-up) with clavicle shaft fractures of greater than 1.5 cm of shortening, each treated nonoperatively (mean shortening 2.3 cm) or with plate fixation (mean shortening 2.5 cm), and found no differences in QuickDASH and Constant shoulder function scores. Furthermore, there were no differences in shoulder range of motion and

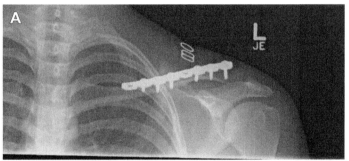
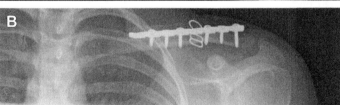
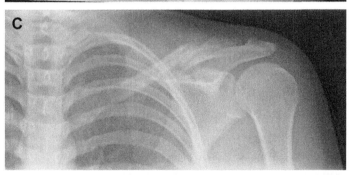
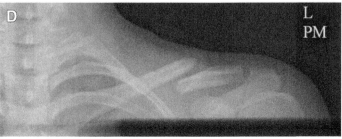

Fig. 3. (A) Anteroposterior (AP) and (B) serendipity radiographs of an 18-year-old female patient status after union of her left clavicle fracture after plate fixation. (C) AP and (D) serendipity radiographs demonstrated a refracture of her left clavicle fracture 4 months after hardware removal from a minor fall off her bicycle.

peak force of the injured extremity when compared with the unaffected extremity in the nonoperative group. The operative group demonstrated slight 3% decrease in abduction peak force in the operated extremity compared with the unaffected extremity though the functional significance of this small difference is unclear. Similarly, Hagstrom and colleagues[27] demonstrated no difference in time to radiographic union, time to return to normal activities, and DASH scores in children with clavicle fractures treated surgically or nonoperatively. However, this study included children as young as 5 years, and the mean age in the 2 groups was different (13.6 years in the operative group and 10.3 years in the nonoperative group). Although these studies had major limitations, they are the first to temper the enthusiasm for surgical treatment by demonstrating that functional outcome regardless of treatment type may be similar in adolescent clavicle fractures.

The question remains about whether malunions in adolescence lead to poor functional outcomes as in adults. Vander Have and colleagues[25] reported that 20% (5 out of 25) of subjects with clavicle fractures treated nonoperatively developed symptomatic malunion, including subjective pain with overhead activity, axillary pain, fatigability, and decreased endurance, though they did not report an objective functional outcome assessment. Bae and colleagues[28] evaluated 16 subjects with clavicle shaft fractures with mean age 12.2 years and greater than 2 cm initial displacement treated nonoperatively with subsequent radiographic malunion, and demonstrated no difference in shoulder abduction and adduction strength compared with the uninjured extremity. They demonstrated slightly reduced forward flexion (7.3°) and abduction (6.5°) compared with the uninjured side after mean 27.2 month follow-up, which is arguably clinically insignificant. Schulz and colleagues[29] also evaluated shoulder functional outcomes in a group of 16 adolescents with midshaft clavicle fractures of more than 100% displacement treated nonoperatively (mean 14.2 years, 2 year follow-up). At final follow-up, there was significant shortening of the injured clavicle, with mean 91.8% length compared with the uninjured clavicle. Despite significant shortening, no subjects had a significant difference in shoulder functional outcome scores, range of motion, and strength between injured and uninjured sides. All subjects in their series also returned to preinjury or higher level of sports participation. The studies by Bae and colleagues,[28] and Schulz and colleagues,[29]

challenge the common belief in the adult literature that shortening and malunion are detrimental to patient function.

Ultimately, there is no high-quality evidence to determine the optimal treatment of clavicle fractures in adolescents. The emerging evidence demonstrating potential equipoise between nonoperative and surgical treatment of adolescent clavicle fractures are predominantly retrospective case series or comparative studies with small sample sizes (Table 1). The largest recent series of adolescent clavicle fractures evaluated 172 subjects who sustained a midshaft clavicle fracture between age 10 to 18 years demonstrated that fracture shortening correlated with poorer Oxford shoulder scores, cosmetic satisfaction scores, and overall satisfaction scores suggesting that malunions may not be benign if a larger sample is studied.[30] For the adult literature to be applied to adolescents, a more detailed analysis of which types of fractures are prone to develop symptomatic malunions in adolescents needs to be reported. Larger sample level I or II evidence will help clarify which adolescent patients can benefit from surgery and which patients need to be treated more like adults. The indications for surgery vary significantly based on the surgeon's interpretation of current literature. In younger adolescents (ages 10–14 years), surgical treatment is reserved for those with severe displacement, though the amount of displacement is arbitrarily determined by the surgeon given that there are no clear guidelines in the literature. The 2 studies evaluating excellent functional outcomes in clavicle malunions in adolescents reported on younger adolescents (mean age 12.2–14.2 years).[28,29] In older adolescents (ages 15–18 years), the investigators generally offer surgery for fractures with greater than 100% superior displacement, greater than 2 cm of initial shortening, as in adults.

ILLUSTRATIVE CASE 1

A 16-year-old male patient sustained a left comminuted clavicle fracture from a dirt bike accident. He underwent a trauma evaluation and did not have any other injuries. Examination of his left shoulder demonstrated no skin tenting or impending open fracture, with a normal neurovascular examination. His radiographs demonstrated superior displacement of the medial fragment with an intermediate segmental comminuted fragment (Fig. 4). Given his older age and the severe amount of displacement, the risks of surgical and nonoperative management were

Table 1 Summary of recent literature in adolescent clavicle fractures						
Study	Design	Number of Subjects in Each Group	Mean Fracture Shortening	Outcomes (Radiographic)	Outcomes (Functional)	Outcomes (Patient-Based)
Vander Have et al,[25] 2010	Retrospective comparative	Nonoperative: 24 Operative: 14 (combined mean age 15.4 y)	Nonoperative: 1.25 cm Operative: 2.75 cm	Mean time to radiographic union Nonoperative: 8.7 wk Operative: 7.4 wk	NA	Mean time to return to activities Nonoperative: 16 wk Operative: 12 wk
Bae et al,[28] 2013	Retrospective case series	Nonoperative: 16 (mean age 12.2 y)	>2 cm inclusion criteria, mean not reported	NA	Compared with contralateral extremity Shoulder range of motion: no difference in all measures except reduced shoulder forward flexion (mean difference 7.3 degrees) and abduction (mean difference 6.5 degrees) in fractured extremity Shoulder strength: no difference in all measures	VAS score for pain: mean 1.6 VAS score for aesthetic satisfaction: mean 2.7 VAS score for satisfaction with treatment: mean 2 DASH score: mean 4.9 PODCI score: mean 97.9

(continued on next page)

Study	Design	Number of Subjects in Each Group	Mean Fracture Shortening	Outcomes (Radiographic)	Outcomes (Functional)	Outcomes (Patient-Based)
Schulz et al,[29] 2013	Retrospective case series	Nonoperative: 16 (mean age 14.2 y)	1.18 cm	% shortening compared with contralateral clavicle AP view: 91.8% Serendipity view: 92.5%	Compared with contralateral extremity Shoulder range of motion: no difference in all measures Shoulder strength: no difference in all measures except external rotation (mean 91.6% compared with contralateral side) Shoulder endurance: no difference in all measures except abduction (mean 88.9% compared with contralateral side)	QuickDASH score: mean 4.5 SANE score: mean 91.1 Constant score: no difference between injured and contralateral side

Study	Design	Number (mean age)	Displacement	Healing	Clinical outcome	Functional scores
Parry et al,[26] 2015	Retrospective comparative	Nonoperative: 8 (mean age 13 y) Operative: 8 (mean age 15 y)	Nonoperative: 2.3 cm Operative: 2.5 cm	NA	Compared with contralateral extremity Shoulder range of motion Nonoperative: no difference in all measures Operative: no difference in all measures Shoulder peak force Nonoperative: no difference in all measures Operative: no difference in all measures except decreased abduction peak force (mean 97% compared with contralateral side)	QuickDASH & Constant scores: perfect (0) except in 1 operative patient
Hagstrom et al,[27] 2015	Retrospective comparative	Nonoperative: 32 (mean age 10.3 y) Operative: 46 (mean age 13.6 y)	>1.5 cm as inclusion mean not reported	Mean time to radiographic healing Nonoperative: 12.02 wk Operative: 11.90 wk (No significant difference)	NA	Mean time to return to activities Nonoperative: 12.24 wk Operative: 12.70 wk (no significant difference) Mean time to full active range of motion Nonoperative: 7.85 wk Operative: 8.74 wk (no significant difference) Mean DASH score Nonoperative: 0.04 Operative: 1.17 (no significant difference)

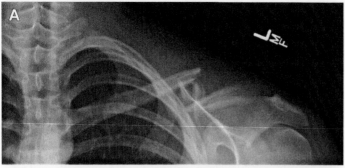
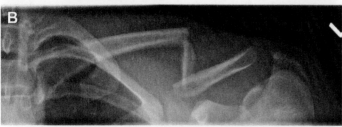
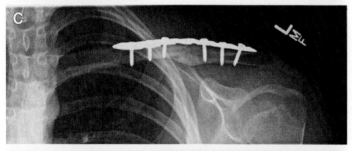
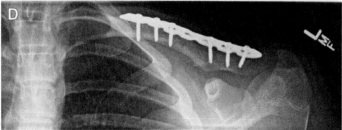

Fig. 4. (A) AP and (B) serendipity radiographs of a 16-year-old male patient with a displaced comminuted left clavicle fracture after a dirt bike accident. (C) AP and (D) serendipity radiographs 10 weeks after open reduction and internal fixation of the fracture.

discussed and the family elected for surgical treatment. Open reduction and internal fixation was performed on his left clavicle with an anatomically contoured superior plate bridging the comminuted fragment. He went on to union by 10 weeks postoperatively, and also achieved full symmetric range of motion by 10 weeks. He returned to baseball by 20 weeks postoperatively and had no pain or sensitivity at the surgical site.

ILLUSTRATIVE CASE 2

A 17-year-old male patient sustained a fall onto his left shoulder while playing football and sustained an isolated left clavicle fracture with 1.5 cm of shortening (Fig. 5), which was treated nonoperatively. He wore a sling full time for 2 weeks and gradually weaned the sling completely by 5 weeks after the injury. He demonstrated radiographic signs of healing by 10 weeks. He returned to playing basketball by 16 weeks and also had no perceivable range of motion deficits noted by the orthopedic surgeon at that time. A final evaluation at 20 weeks postinjury demonstrated full radiographic healing, a painless palpable bump at the fracture site, return to full sporting activities, and complete patient satisfaction with his outcome.

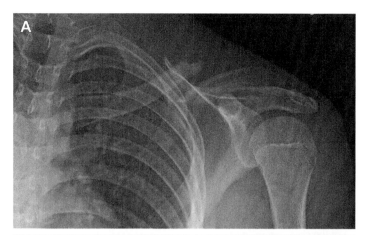
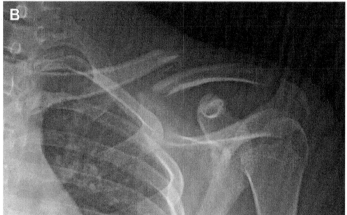
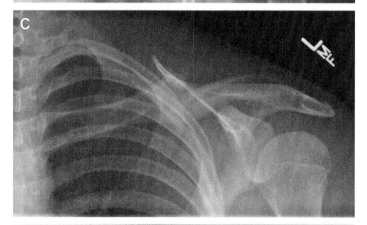
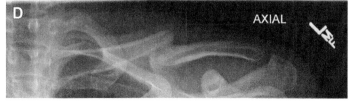

Fig. 5. (A) AP and (B) serendipity radiographs of a 17-year-old male patient with a 1.5 cm shortened left clavicle fracture after a football injury. (C) AP and (D) serendipity radiographs 20 weeks after nonoperative treatment.

REFERENCES

1. Caird MS. Clavicle shaft fractures: are children little adults? J Pediatr Orthop 2012;32(Suppl 1):S1–4.
2. Anwar I, Amiras D, Khanna M, et al. Physes around the shoulder girdle: normal development and injury patterns. Clin Radiol 2016;71(7):702–9.
3. McGraw MA, Mehlman CT, Lindsell CJ, et al. Postnatal growth of the clavicle: birth to 18 years of age. J Pediatr Orthop 2009;29(8):937–43.
4. Lenza M, Belloti JC, Andriolo RB, et al. Conservative interventions for treating middle third clavicle fractures in adolescents and adults. Cochrane Database Syst Rev 2014;(5):CD007121.
5. Neviaser RJ, Neviaser JS, Neviaser TJ, et al. A simple technique for internal fixation of the clavicle. A long term evaluation. Clin Orthop Relat Res 1975;(109):103–7.
6. Grassi FA, Tajana MS, D'Angelo F. Management of midclavicular fractures: comparison between nonoperative treatment and open intramedullary fixation in 80 patients. J Trauma 2001;50(6):1096–100.
7. Houwert RM, Wijdicks FJ, Steins Bisschop C, et al. Plate fixation versus intramedullary fixation for displaced mid-shaft clavicle fractures: a systematic review. Int Orthop 2012;36(3):579–85.
8. Strauss EJ, Egol KA, France MA, et al. Complications of intramedullary Hagie pin fixation for acute midshaft clavicle fractures. J Shoulder Elbow Surg 2007;16(3):280–4.
9. Naimark M, Dufka FL, Han R, et al. Plate fixation of midshaft clavicular fractures: patient-reported outcomes and hardware-related complications. J Shoulder Elbow Surg 2016;25(5):739–46.
10. Canadian Orthopaedic Trauma Society. Nonoperative treatment compared with plate fixation of displaced midshaft clavicular fractures. A multicenter, randomized clinical trial. J Bone Joint Surg Am 2007;89(1):1–10.
11. Hill JM, McGuire MH, Crosby LA. Closed treatment of displaced middle-third fractures of the clavicle gives poor results. J Bone Joint Surg Br 1997; 79(4):537–9.
12. McKee MD, Pedersen EM, Jones C, et al. Deficits following nonoperative treatment of displaced midshaft clavicular fractures. J Bone Joint Surg Am 2006;88(1):35–40.
13. Nowak J, Holgersson M, Larsson S. Sequelae from clavicular fractures are common: a prospective study of 222 patients. Acta Orthop 2005;76(4):496–502.
14. Wick M, Muller EJ, Kollig E, et al. Midshaft fractures of the clavicle with a shortening of more than 2 cm predispose to nonunion. Arch Orthop Trauma Surg 2001;121(4):207–11.
15. Potter JM, Jones C, Wild LM, et al. Does delay matter? The restoration of objectively measured shoulder strength and patient-oriented outcome after immediate fixation versus delayed reconstruction of displaced midshaft fractures of the clavicle. J Shoulder Elbow Surg 2007;16(5):514–8.
16. Yang S, Werner BC, Gwathmey FW Jr. Treatment trends in adolescent clavicle fractures. J Pediatr Orthop 2015;35(3):229–33.
17. Robinson CM, Court-Brown CM, McQueen MM, et al. Estimating the risk of nonunion following nonoperative treatment of a clavicular fracture. J Bone Joint Surg Am 2004;86-A(7):1359–65.
18. Robinson CM, Goudie EB, Murray IR, et al. Open reduction and plate fixation versus nonoperative treatment for displaced midshaft clavicular fractures: a multicenter, randomized, controlled trial. J Bone Joint Surg Am 2013;95(17):1576–84.
19. Pourtaheri N, Strongwater AM. Clavicle nonunion in a 10-year-old boy. Orthopedics 2012;35(3):e442–3.
20. Caterini R, Farsetti P, Barletta V. Posttraumatic nonunion of the clavicle in a 7-year-old girl. Arch Orthop Trauma Surg 1998;117(8):475–6.
21. Ropars M, Bey M, Bouin M, et al. Posttraumatic nonunion of the clavicle in a child: case report. Rev Chir Orthop Reparatrice Appar Mot 2004; 90(7):666–9.
22. Spapens N, Degreef I, Debeer P. Posttraumatic pseudarthrosis of the clavicle in an 8-year-old girl. J Pediatr Orthop B 2010;19(2):188–90.
23. Mehlman CT, Yihua G, Bochang C, et al. Operative treatment of completely displaced clavicle shaft fractures in children. J Pediatr Orthop 2009;29(8):851–5.
24. Namdari S, Ganley TJ, Baldwin K, et al. Fixation of displaced midshaft clavicle fractures in skeletally immature patients. J Pediatr Orthop 2011;31(5):507–11.
25. Vander Have KL, Perdue AM, Caird MS, et al. Operative versus nonoperative treatment of midshaft clavicle fractures in adolescents. J Pediatr Orthop 2010;30(4):307–12.
26. Parry JA, Van Straaten M, Luo TD, et al. Is there a deficit after nonoperative versus operative treatment of shortened midshaft clavicular fractures in adolescents? J Pediatr Orthop 2015. [Epub ahead of print].
27. Hagstrom LS, Ferrick M, Galpin R. Outcomes of operative versus nonoperative treatment of displaced pediatric clavicle fractures. Orthopedics 2015;38(2):e135–8.
28. Bae DS, Shah AS, Kalish LA, et al. Shoulder motion, strength, and functional outcomes in children with established malunion of the clavicle. J Pediatr Orthop 2013;33(5):544–50.
29. Schulz J, Moor M, Roocroft J, et al. Functional and radiographic outcomes of nonoperative treatment of displaced adolescent clavicle fractures. J Bone Joint Surg Am 2013;95(13):1159–65.
30. Randsborg PH, Fuglesang HF, Røtterud JH, et al. Long-term patient-reported outcome after fractures of the clavicle in patients aged 10 to 18 years. J Pediatr Orthop 2014;34(4):393–9.

Complications of Pediatric Foot and Ankle Fractures

Jaime R. Denning, MD

KEYWORDS

- Pediatric foot and ankle fractures • Complications • Premature physeal closure
- Posttraumatic arthritis

KEY POINTS

- Phalangeal fractures that are at the highest risk for complications include intraarticular phalangeal fractures of the hallux, distal phalangeal physeal fractures that extend through the nail matrix, and phalangeal fractures with severe flexion/extension displacement.
- Foot fractures that are at the highest risk for complications include Jones fifth metatarsal fractures, Lisfranc, talus, and calcaneus fractures.
- Ankle fractures that are at the highest risk for complications include high-energy fractures, articular displacement greater than 2 mm or physeal widening greater than 3 mm after final reduction.
- Children with chronic regional pain syndrome type I (CRPSI) have a higher preponderance of foot and ankle injuries than adults with CRPSI.

INTRODUCTION

Ankle fractures account for 5% and foot fractures account for approximately 8% of fractures in children.[1,2] Although there is abundant literature discussing adult treatment and outcomes (including complications) of foot and ankle trauma, there is a paucity of literature specifically discussing certain risks and treatments of ankle, and especially foot, injuries in children. Some complications, including compartment syndrome (CS), extensor retinaculum syndrome, reflex sympathetic dystrophy (RSD)/complex regional pain syndrome, infection, neurovascular injuries, and cast complications, are evident early in the treatment or natural history of foot and ankle fractures. Other complications, such as osteonecrosis (ON), missed injuries, premature physeal closure (PPC), malunion, nonunion, and arthrofibrosis, do not become apparent until weeks, months, or years after the original fracture. The incidence of long-term sequelae like posttraumatic arthritis from childhood foot and ankle fractures is poorly studied because decades or lifelong follow-up have not been accomplished to date. This article discusses a variety of complications associated with foot and ankle fractures in children or the treatment of these injuries. Foot fractures, including those of the phalanges, metatarsals, Lisfranc complex, talus, and calcaneus, and pediatric ankle fractures, including physeal, triplane, and Tillaux fractures, are described with a brief overview of each type followed by the complications unique to each fracture type. General complications associated with any pediatric foot or ankle injury are reviewed at the end of the article.

FOOT INJURIES

Phalangeal Fractures

The incidence of phalangeal fractures in children is not reported in the literature. The mechanism of injury is usually a stubbing injury or an object dropped on the toe. There have been a few recent case series specifically discussing skeletally immature patients with intraarticular hallux phalangeal fractures.[3,4]

The generally accepted threshold for choosing operative fixation of an intraarticular

Orthopaedic Surgery, Cincinnati Children's Hospital Medical Center, 3333 Burnet Avenue, ML 2017, Cincinnati, OH 45229, USA
E-mail address: jaime.denning@cchmc.org

Orthop Clin N Am 48 (2017) 59–70
http://dx.doi.org/10.1016/j.ocl.2016.08.010
0030-5898/17/© 2016 Elsevier Inc. All rights reserved.

proximal phalanx fracture of the hallux is involvement of more than 30% of the articular surface or articular displacement greater than 3 mm.[5,6]

To avoid certain phalangeal fracture complications (even rare ones), treating providers should not always just assume that all toes fractures in children will do well. The phalangeal fractures listed in Table 1 (and discussed later) should be approached with appropriate caution.

Posttraumatic arthritis/hallux rigidus

Damaging any joint (intraarticular injury) increases the chances of developing arthritis 7-fold, according to the American Academy of Orthopaedic Surgeons (AAOS).[7] Kramer and colleagues[4] reported on a series of 10 patients with intraarticular hallux fractures occurring at an average age of 12.6 years, who were followed for a median 50.5 months (longest follow-up was 123 months); there was a 10% rate of posttraumatic arthritis requiring fusion.

Infection

Pinckney fractures are distal phalangeal physeal fractures that extend through the nail matrix. These fractures usually occur in the hallux. If they are not recognized or treated appropriately as open fractures, osteomyelitis can occur. In Pinckney and colleagues'[8] original article describing this injury in 6 children, the first 4 presented with cellulitis or osteomyelitis, but the last 2 were given antibiotics and did not develop infection caused by this open fracture type. To minimize the infection risk, treatment can be extrapolated from the hand literature describing appropriate treatment of Seymour fractures, Salter-Harris (SH) I or II fractures of the distal phalanx of the hand with associated nailbed laceration. Timely (within 24 hours) treatment involves irrigation and debridement, fracture reduction to ensure that there is no interposed periosteum in the fracture site, and antibiotic administration.[9] In the study by Reyes and Ho,[9] there were 0 out of 11 infections in the group treated within 24 hours of sustaining a Seymour fracture, and there were 5 out of 11 (45%) infections in the delayed treatment group.

Rare phalangeal fracture complications

Phalangeal fractures in children can, rarely, result in ON and malunion. ON is a rare complication of intraarticular hallux phalangeal fractures that usually occurs if there is disruption of the vascularity of small fragments attached to the collateral ligament.[4] Fig. 1 shows an example of ON of a phalangeal fracture treated with open reduction with Kirschner (K) wire fixation. Phalangeal fractures (except border toes) can tolerate some varus/valgus and rotation, but can create abnormal pressure/callus on the plantar surface of the foot or difficulty with shoe wear if they heal in flexion or extension. Fig. 2 shows a case that could have healed in excessive extension if treated without reduction and fixation.

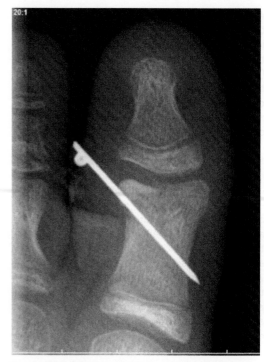

Fig. 1. ON of the lateral distal aspect of a hallux proximal phalangeal fracture treated with open reduction and Kirschner-wire fixation. Soft tissue stripping of the tiny fragment at the time of open reduction likely caused this ON, which did not cause any pain to the patient once the fracture healed.

Table 1 Phalangeal fractures in children with high risk of complications	
Type of Phalangeal Fracture	**Complication**
Intra-articular phalangeal fractures of hallux	Posttraumatic arthritis
Distal phalangeal physeal fractures that extend through nail matrix (Pinckney fracture)	Infection
Phalangeal fracture with severe flexion/extension displacement	Malunion

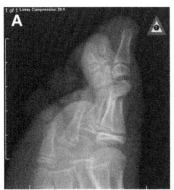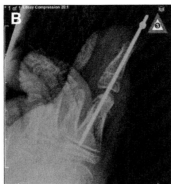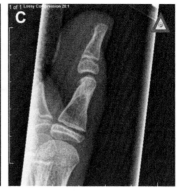

Fig. 2. (A) Hallux proximal phalangeal neck fracture with nearly 90° extension deformity, (B) after open reduction and pinning of the fracture, and (C) after hardware removal and uneventful healing of the fracture.

Metatarsal Fractures

A British epidemiologic study of pediatric fractures showed that the incidence of foot fractures was 10.5 per 10,000 children less than 18 years old and that they occurred most commonly in both boys and girls around age 13 years.[2] Metatarsal fractures in children account for 60% to 90% of pediatric foot fractures.[5,10] Foot fractures at high risk for complications are discussed later and in Table 2.

Nonunion

Similar to adults, the most common site of metatarsal fracture nonunion in children is the proximal metaphyseal-diaphyseal junction of the fifth metatarsal (Jones fracture). Risk of nonunion at this site is most common in children more than 13 years of age and in patients with preceding stress injury indicated by pain at that site before traumatic injury.[11] Knowledge of which patients are at highest risk of nonunion with nonoperative cast treatment can expedite operative treatment with an intramedullary screw when indicated.

Fig. 3 shows an example of a healthy 10-year-old girl with painful nonunion of her fifth metatarsal base Jones fracture, which failed multiple attempts at both non–weight-bearing and weight-bearing cast immobilization before having successful union after open reduction and internal fixation (ORIF) with a cannulated screw.

Compartment syndrome of the foot

High-energy crush injuries to the foot with or without multiple foot fractures can result in excessive swelling within the 9 compartments of the foot. CS presents differently in children than in adults; usually an increasing analgesia requirement is the primary sign. It is also harder to differentiate between direct foot injury pain and foot CS pain, whereas foot symptoms that indicate a CS with a more proximal injury such as a tibia fracture are at least easier to differentiate. There should be a low threshold in children to check compartment pressure measurements, usually under anesthesia. Measurements of any compartment greater than 30 mm Hg or less than 30 mm Hg less than patient's diastolic blood pressure are the accepted thresholds for performing fasciotomies through 2 dorsal longitudinal incisions and a medial incision along the arch.[12] The most sensitive of the 9 compartments for measuring compartment pressures is the calcaneal compartment.[13] The incidence of pediatric foot CS is unknown, but a recent article by Wallin and colleagues[14] included a systematic literature review from 1990 to 2012 and found 8 studies, including 59 pediatric patients between the ages of 1.5 and 18 years, with traumatic foot CS. There were not many long-term outcomes presented in these studies, but a follow-up study of 7 pediatric patients treated with fasciotomies for foot CS for an average of 41 months all had good or excellent results.[15] Late sequelae of

Table 2
Foot fractures in children with high risk of complications

Type of Foot Fracture	Complication
Jones fracture (metaphyseal-diaphyseal fifth metatarsal fracture)	Nonunion
Lisfranc fracture	Arthritis
Talus fracture	ON, concurrent injury, OCD
Calcaneal fracture	Associated injury, arthritis

Abbreviation: OCD, osteochondral defect.

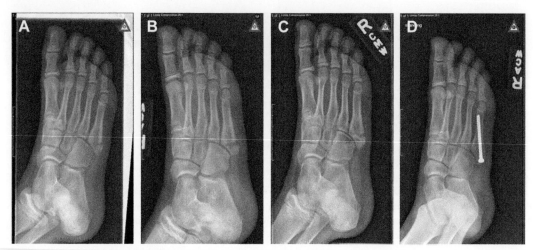

Fig. 3. Ten-year-old girl with painful nonunion of her fifth metatarsal base Jones fracture at the time of injury (*A*), and after 1 month of weight bearing as tolerated in a below-knee cast (*B*). Patient was still tender at fracture site 3 months later after non–weight bearing with a cast then a boot (*C*). Successful union occurred 6 weeks after open reduction and internal fixation with a cannulated screw. One-year follow-up showed complete healing and no hardware complications (*D*).

missed foot CS reported in different a publication include pain, claw toes, paresthesias, and cavus foot.[16]

Lisfranc Fractures

In adults, Lisfranc injuries account for less than 1% of all fractures.[17] Lisfranc injuries are even more rare in children and the patients tend to do well.[18–20] The largest published case series of pediatric Lisfranc injuries comprises 18 patients 16 years old and younger (average age 12 years) with a range of injuries from mild displacement to frank tarsometatarsal (TMT) joint dislocation. The most common mechanism of injury was falling with the foot in equinus position and the fractures in this series were treated very differently from the standard adult treatment of ORIF or primary TMT arthrodesis. Most were treated with closed reduction and casting or closed reduction and K-wire fixation, 14 out of 18 patients were asymptomatic at final follow-up 3 to 8 months after injury, and 4 out of 18 patients had only minor pain 1 year postinjury.[18] In a series of 41 patients with pediatric Lisfranc (average age, 11 + 4 years), 13 of whom completed outcomes questionnaires an average of 5 years after injury, nonoperative treatment resulted in excellent long-term function and quality of life. Operative treatment was performed in older patients (>12 years old) with more complicated and displaced injuries and resulted in worse but still good function and quality of life.[20] The preferred method of treatment of Lisfranc injuries in children is unclear, but most Lisfranc injuries in children, especially those less than 12 years of age, are treated nonoperatively with a short-leg cast for about a month.[18–20]

Malunion/posttraumatic arthritis

In the Wiley[18] study, 2 out of 18 patients had angular deformity (malunion) from incomplete reduction, but long-term follow-up was lacking so the rate of posttraumatic arthritis is unknown. In the Buoncristiani and colleagues[19] study, one of the 8 patients in the series had radiograph evidence of arthritis across the TMT joint at 39 months after Lisfranc injury and the investigators concluded that the patient should have been treated with ORIF instead of short-leg casting alone. In the Denning and colleagues[20] study, 21% of patients had residual angulation, displacement, or malunion and 38% of patients had radiographic evidence of TMT and/or other midfoot arthritis at final radiographic follow-up. The rates of malunion and arthritis were not significantly different between operatively and nonoperatively treated groups.[20]

Missed injury

The rate of missed Lisfranc injuries in children is unknown, but in the adult literature up to 20% of these injuries are missed on initial anteroposterior (AP) and lateral radiographs.[17,21] Weight-bearing radiographs should be performed if there is suspicion of a Lisfranc injury and initial injury films do not show any injury. MRI is capable of showing ligamentous tears if the radiographs are inconclusive.

Talus Fractures

Talus fractures account for less than 0.1% of all pediatric fractures, which makes them more rare than adult talus fractures, which make up 0.3% of fractures.[5] In biomechanical studies, it takes nearly twice the force to fracture a child's talus than to fracture the ankle or other tarsal bones.[22] The usual mechanism of injury is a fall from a height with the ankle in forced dorsiflexion.

Osteonecrosis

In the pediatric population, the rate of ON is lower than that of adults with talus fractures in some studies.[23] Other studies conclude that the ON rate in children with talus fractures equals or exceeds that of adults.[24] From the literature review in the Rammelt and colleagues[24] article, there was a 16% incidence of ON in nondisplaced talus fractures in children. Half of the fractures going on to ON were initially missed on radiograph at the time of injury and all of the children with these nondisplaced fractures that went on to ON were less than 9 years old. The Hawkins sign is a radiographic finding of subchondral lucency that occurs by 1 to 2 months postinjury and indicates adequate blood flow to the talar body following talus fracture in adults.[25] Ogden[26] suggests that the Hawkins sign is not reliable in children because the talar dome is cartilaginous. The Hawkins classification is a classification system from I to IV based on degree of displacement of the talar neck fracture, and, although it bears the same name, is different from the Hawkins sign described earlier. This classification system is predictive of ON rate in adults, but it does not correlate in with risk of ON in children. The literature regarding children with talar fractures indicates that ON seems to be unpredictable, so the treating clinician should follow children closely after all talus fractures, including nondisplaced injuries.

Posttraumatic arthritis

Because much of the talus is covered in articular cartilage, the rule of striving for anatomic reduction of an intraarticular fracture is applicable in 3 separate joints during talus fracture reduction: the tibiotalar, subtalar, and talonavicular joints. Posttraumatic arthritis occurred in 3 out of 12 patients in a study with an average 11-year follow-up after pediatric talus fractures. One patient had to be treated with pantalar arthrodesis and 2 patients with ankle arthrodesis. The average American Orthopedic Foot and Ankle Society (AOFAS) ankle-hindfoot score at 1 to 22 years postinjury was 85 (range, 65–100).[27]

Talar malunion

The most common malunion either from incomplete reduction or loss of fixation after surgical treatment of talus fractures is hindfoot varus malalignment and forefoot adduction and supination from medial column shortening. Subtalar joint incongruity is also common. Even in pediatric patients, the remodeling potential of the talus is not good.[28]

Concurrent injury

Because talus fractures tend to be high-energy injuries, concurrent injuries with talus fractures in children are common. To prevent the possibility of a missed injury, treating providers should have a high index of suspicion to look for concomitant injuries with talar fractures. In the Meier and colleagues[27] study, there were 7 out of 15 pediatric patients with talus fracture with concurrent injuries to the same extremity and 4 of those patients had more than 1 associated injury. Fig. 4 shows an example of a skeletally immature patient with talar neck fracture/dislocation with concurrent medial and lateral malleolus fractures.

Osteochondral fracture

Osteochondral lesions of the talus are sequelae of talar trauma, although the accepted rate varies widely in the literature from 47% to 80% of osteochondral lesions thought to be caused by preceding trauma.[29,30] Lateral osteochondral lesions are more commonly from trauma than medial lesions, which are often caused by repetitive stress/microtrauma. To prevent missing a small osteochondral lesion, treating providers should consider standard AP, mortise, and lateral ankle radiographs, plus oblique and plantar flexion radiographs or MRI if pain and swelling of the ankle joint persist more than 2 months after talar fracture.

Calcaneus Fractures

Calcaneus fractures in children are rare; there is no reported incidence in the literature because only case reports and small series are available. In a long-term follow-up (mean 16.8 years after injury) of 17 patients less than 14 years of age when they sustained 19 calcaneal fractures, the outcomes were excellent (AOFAS ankle-hindfoot average score 96.2 out of 100) after cast treatment in all but 1 patient who had an open fracture.[31] In older adolescents or children with severely displaced fractures, operative reduction and fixation should be considered, including closed reduction and percutaneous fixation.[32,33]

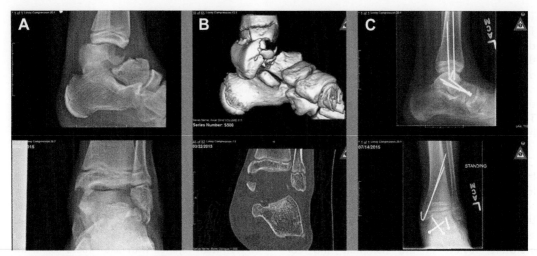

Fig. 4. A skeletally immature patient with talar neck fracture/dislocation with concurrent medial and lateral malleolus fractures on plain films (*A*), computed tomography (*B*), and after open reduction and internal fixation (*C*). There is no obvious ON seen on postoperative films.

Associated injuries

In a study of 56 calcaneus fractures in children, Schmidt and Weiner[34] found that associated injuries were more common when the patients were more than 13 years of age and that lower extremity concomitant fractures were twice as common as in adults, but axial skeleton concomitant injuries were less common than in adults. In Brunet's[31] study of 17 children with 19 calcaneal fractures, there were 5 ipsilateral foot fractures, including talar neck, Lisfranc, and cuneiform fractures. In Wiley and Profitt's[35] study of 32 children with calcaneal fractures, associated injuries were less common, with only 2 out of 32 having a concomitant injury.

Wound/skin complications

Wound complications were less common in pediatric patients treated with ORIF of their calcaneus fractures than in adults undergoing ORIF. This finding is likely attributable to children having fewer risk factors/comorbidities that predispose to lower extremity wound complications. In a small sample size, Pickle and colleagues[36] had 0 out of 6 wound complications in pediatric patients who underwent ORIF calcaneus fracture. This finding compares with a reported 25% rate of wound complications after adult calcaneus ORIF. In a direct comparison study between pediatric and adult calcaneal fractures treated with ORIF at Harborview, there were 0 out of 21 pediatric calcanei with wound complications and 7 out of 368 (2%) adults with wound healing problems.[37]

ANKLE INJURIES

Ankle Fractures, Including Triplane/Tillaux Transitional Fractures

Ankle fractures in children make up approximately 5% of pediatric fractures.[1] Pediatric ankle fractures account for 9% to 18% of all growth plate fractures.[38] Pediatric patients with ankle fractures who have more than 2 years of growth remaining generally have satisfactory outcomes after restoration of joint line alignment and preservation of physeal growth.[1] Transitional fractures of the distal tibia are specific fractures caused by a partially closed and partially open distal tibial physis. The pattern of distal tibial physeal closure begins centrally and extends medially and then laterally; this process takes about 18 months to complete and it is during this time that the asymmetric physeal closure is responsible for Tillaux and triplane fracture patterns.[6] Tillaux fractures are caused by an avulsion of the anterolateral tibial epiphysis by the anterior-inferior tibiofibular ligament via an external rotation mechanism. Triplane fractures are 2-part, 3-part, or 4-part fractures that occur in sagittal, coronal, and transverse planes and about half of triplane fractures have an associated fibular fracture.[38] The mean age at the time of triplane fracture was 12.8 years for girls and 14.8 years for boys.[39] Computed tomography scans are useful for classification and surgical planning of these injuries.[40] In a study of 237 pediatric patients with distal tibia and fibula fractures, Tillaux fractures occurred in 2.9% and triplane fractures in 7.3%.[41] Indication for surgical treatment is inability to achieve less than

2 mm of articular displacement or less than 3 mm of physeal displacement by closed means.[1,38]

Premature physeal closure

Risk of PPC after distal tibia physeal fracture is highest after SH III and IV fractures (7%–38%), then SH I and II fractures (2%–38%).[1,41,42] Clinically relevant PPC after triplane and Tillaux fractures is rare because patients tend to be closer to skeletal maturity at the time of these injuries, and articular displacement is more of a concern.[41] Risk of PPC does not seem to be affected by number of reduction attempts of physeal fractures, initial displacement of the fracture, or method of treatment.[1,43] Lack of an associated fibula fracture with distal tibia physeal fractures/triplane fractures had a positive influence on fracture outcome (less PPC).[44,45] Barmada and colleagues'[1] study of 92 distal tibia physeal fractures showed that, in SH I and II fractures, PPC risk was 60% if physeal widening was greater than 3 mm after final reduction and 17% in patients with less than 3 mm widening. Fig. 5 shows an example of an 11-year-old boy with an SH II distal tibia fracture that could not be adequately reduced closed. The mechanism of injury also seems to influence the risk of PPC; supination–external rotation injuries resulted in PPC 35% of the time and pronation-abduction injuries 54% of the time.[46] PPC after distal tibia physeal fracture can result in angular deformity, most commonly distal tibial varus.[47] Angular deformity is most common after a high-energy mechanism of injury. In a study of 24 patients with distal tibia growth disturbance, 13 out of 15 high-energy fractures resulted in angular deformity compared with 1 out of 9 low-energy fractures resulting in angular deformity.[48] PPC can also result in angular deformity from tibia/fibula growth mismatch. If the fibula continues to grow after a tibial growth arrest, the patient can get fibula/calcaneus abutment when the hindfoot is everted. In contrast, if the tibia continues to grow after distal fibula arrest, the ankle can grow into valgus alignment. Rarely, PPC of the distal tibia can result in clinically significant leg length discrepancy if the fracture occurs when the patient has several years of growth remaining. The anatomic location of PPC in the distal tibia involved the anteromedial physis in 65% of cases (the site of earliest physiologic closure of the physis) in an MRI study.[49] Treatment of patients with PPC includes physeal bar resection for less than 50% of the physis, epiphysiodesis, and osteotomies.[50] Box 1 provides a summary of the ankle fractures at highest risk for PPC.

Malunion

Rotational malunions do not remodel the way frontal and sagittal plane deformities can in a growing child. External rotation of the distal tibia causing external foot progression angle

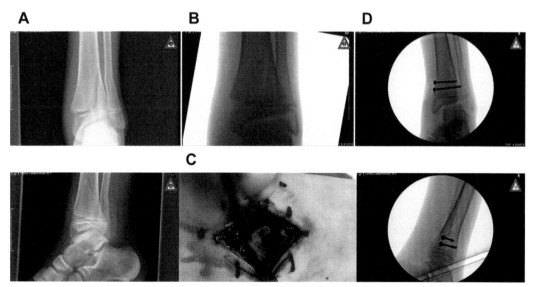

Fig. 5. (A) Eleven-year-old boy with SH II distal tibia fracture on AP and lateral radiographs. (B) After attempted closed reduction under general anesthetic, the fracture alignment still had significant rotational and physeal displacement. (C) Clinical view of the patient's physis with a large flap of periosteum held up by forceps that had been blocking the reduction. (D) Final fluoroscopic images of the fracture after open reduction and screw fixation.

Box 1
Ankle fractures at high risk for PPC

SH III/IV > SH I/II > triplane > Tillaux

Associated fibula fracture

SH I/II with pronation-abduction mechanism > supination–external rotation mechanism

High-energy mechanism of injury

SH I/II with physeal widening >3 mm after final reduction

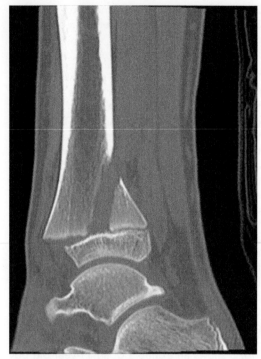

Fig. 6. Lateral ankle computed tomography view of a 15-year-old boy with SH II distal tibia fracture with extreme pain, weakness of his EHL, and first dorsal web space paresthesias. The sharp, unreduced metaphyseal prominence can be seen compressing the structures anterior to it, causing the symptoms of extensor retinaculum syndrome. His symptoms resolved completely after open reduction and fixation of his fracture.

can result from distal tibia SH I or II or triplane fracture malunions.[51,52] Surgical treatment of distal tibia malunions ranges from hemiepiphysiodesis in skeletally immature patients with angular deformity in 1 plane to osteotomies for patients with rotational deformity or skeletally mature patients with angular deformity.

Missed fracture
In 215 patients with foot fractures during retrospective evaluation of their radiographs, there were concurrent unrecognized fractures of the distal tibia and fibula in 8%.[53] Treating providers should also have a high index of suspicion for a more proximal tibia fracture in patients with a triplane fracture; an 8.5% rate of tibial shaft fractures was found in a series of patients with triplane fracture and cases of Maissoneuve-type proximal fibula fractures have been reported.[38,54]

Extensor retinaculum syndrome
Mubarak[55] described extensor retinaculum syndrome in 6 patients with severe pain and swelling, decreased sensation in the first web space, weakness of extensor hallucis longus (EHL) and extensor digitorum longus, and pain with passive flexion of toes. This entity is separate from CS of the anterior compartment and usually involves a displaced triplane fracture with the anterior metaphyseal spike compressing the muscle bellies of extensor hallucis and peroneus tertius and deep peroneal nerve against the underside of the rigid superior extensor retinaculum. Time from injury to reduction of the fracture averaged 25 hours in Mubarak's[55] study, so delay in reduction seems to play a role in development of superior retinaculum syndrome. Fig. 6 shows a lateral ankle computed tomography view of a 15-year-old boy who sustained a SH II distal tibia fracture and had an unsuccessful reduction with excruciating pain, weakness of his EHL, and first dorsal web space paresthesias. Diagnosis of this condition is mostly clinical and measuring increased compartment pressure within the extensor retinaculum confirms the diagnosis. There is no absolute value for what pressure reading constitutes an extensor retinaculum syndrome. The treatment of this complication is prompt reduction of the fracture and surgical release of the superior retinaculum.

Chronic regional pain syndrome type I/reflex sympathetic dystrophy
CRPSI was previously called RSD and is not a result of a direct peripheral nerve injury. CRPSI has diagnostic criteria including pain out of proportion to inciting event and some or all of the following associated symptoms: sensory, vasomotor, sweating, edema, motor, or trophic changes. Children with CRPSI have a higher preponderance of lower extremity injuries than adults. In a group of 70 children treated for CRPSI, 87% had a lower extremity injury as the inciting event.[56] In a study of 24 children with CRPSI, 73% had specifically foot or ankle

injuries.[57] Girls are more commonly affected than boys (84%) and average age of onset is 12.5 years.[56] Diagnosis of CRPSI remains difficult and children often experience symptoms for 9 to 12 months before definitive diagnosis is made and treatment begins.[58,59] In addition to using clinical findings of pain, dysesthesia, and autonomic instability, a specific finding called tache cérébrale is a helpful sign of vasomotor dysfunction.[58] Tache cérébrale is when a fingernail drawn across the patient's affected skin causes a red line to appear shortly thereafter. Treatment ranges from outpatient massage and mobilization to multidisciplinary inpatient regimens with involvement of anesthesia pain, orthopedic surgery, physical medicine, psychiatry, and physical therapy teams.[60] Children respond better to physical therapy and noninvasive treatments than adults, but recur more often.[59] Although children have reportedly had better outcomes after CRPSI than adults, 54% of children in multidisciplinary treatment programs still have some CRPSI symptoms 3 years after diagnosis.[56] In an adult follow-up study of 42 patients who had CRPSI during childhood/adolescence (mean 12-year follow-up), 52% still had pain in the affected limb.[61] Fig. 7 shows radiographic studies of an 11.5-year-old premenarchal girl who sustained a triplane fracture and experienced CRPSI both during the initial postinjury period and during the postsurgical period 1 year later when she had to undergo epiphysiodesis for growth arrest of her distal tibia, which was causing angular deformity.

Degenerative changes/posttraumatic arthritis

The goal of intraarticular ankle fracture treatment is to restore anatomic alignment of the joint line, although accomplishing this via operative or nonoperative means does not guarantee that arthritis will not occur. In a long-term study of 68 patients (62 of whom were treated nonoperatively) followed for an average of 27 years postinjury, there was a nearly 12% rate of radiographic osteoarthritis and pain.[62] All but 1 of these patients with osteoarthritis on radiographs had SH III or IV fractures as children. In a study of 23 patients with triplane fracture, 50% of patients reported pain 3 to 13 years after the ankle injury.[63] Having greater than 2 mm of residual displacement in the weight-bearing zone of the distal tibia or 10° of distal tibia angular deformity was associated with increased ankle joint stress and less favorable outcomes.[38,64] Table 3 lists ankle fractures associated with high rates of complications.

GENERAL COMPLICATIONS

Other complications to consider in association with foot and ankle fractures are venous thromboembolism (VTE), skin complications, and other cast-associated complications. VTE is extremely rare in pediatric lower extremity trauma (0.058% incidence) and foot and ankle injuries specifically made up only 18.5% of the lower extremity injuries that had concurrent VTE in a large retrospective database study.[65] Cast complications can range from skin blisters and ulceration to cast saw burns at the time of cast removal to osteopenia from immobilization. In adolescents with lower extremity fractures immobilized in casts, the bone mineral density on the fractured leg compared with the uninjured leg at the time of cast removal ranged from −5.8% to −31.7%.[66] Recovery time to normal bone mineral density is unknown and thus a theoretic risk of

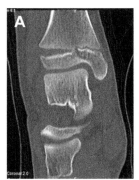 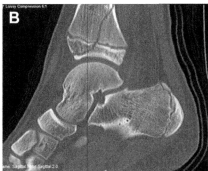 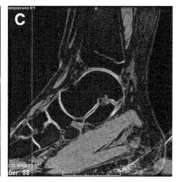

Fig. 7. (A, B) Computed tomography scan at the time of original injury to 11.5-year-old girl who sustained a triplane fracture and experienced CRPSI both during the initial postinjury period when she was treated with non-weight bearing cast immobilization and during the postsurgical period 1 year later when she had to undergo epiphysiodesis for growth arrest of her distal tibia. (C) MRI of her partial growth arrest.

Table 3
Ankle fracture types associated with higher rates of complications

Type of Ankle Fracture or Patient	Complications
Girl, around 12 y old, pain out of proportion to foot or ankle fracture/injury	CRPSI
Triplane or displaced SH II (especially delayed reduction)	Extensor retinaculum syndrome, associated tibia shaft fracture
>2 mm articular displacement	Arthritis
>10° distal tibia angular deformity	Arthritis

repeat fracture to the same limb exists. Skin complications secondary to swelling include fracture blisters and fasciotomy scars. Open fractures and lawnmower or degloving injuries can also cause skin complications.

SUMMARY

Children with operative and nonoperative treatment of foot and ankle fractures generally do well. Providers who care for these children should keep the following high-risk fracture types and parameters in mind to prevent complications in these patients. Intraarticular hallux phalangeal fractures with 30% articular involvement or greater than 3 mm of displacement and phalangeal fractures with severe flexion/extension should be reduced and stabilized appropriately. Distal phalangeal physeal fractures that extend through the nail matrix should be irrigated/debrided, reduced without interposed tissue, and given antibiotics. Jones fifth metatarsal fractures should be followed closely for delayed or nonunion. Lisfranc, talus, and calcaneus fractures are rare in children, but, when they occur, clinicians should be aware of possible concurrent injuries and future complications, such as ON and arthritis. Pediatric ankle fractures should have articular displacement reduced to less than 2 mm of separation and physeal widening reduced to less than 3 mm of displacement to avoid future arthritis or physeal arrest. Providers who treat pediatric foot and ankle fractures should consider diagnosis of CRPSI in patients whose pain is out of proportion to the severity of injury or in whom pain persists for longer than anticipated after radiographic healing. More studies are needed to show the long-term outcomes after pediatric foot and ankle trauma.

REFERENCES

1. Barmada A, Gaynor T, Mubarak SJ. Premature physeal closure following distal tibia physeal fractures: a new radiographic predictor. J Pediatr Orthop 2003;32(6):733–9.
2. Cooper C, Dennison EM, Leufkens HGM, et al. Epidemiology of childhood fractures in Britain: a study using the general practice research database. J Bone Miner Res 2004;19(12):1976–81.
3. Bariteau JT, Murillo DM, Tenenbaum SA, et al. Joint salvage after neglected intra-articular physeal fracture of the hallux in high-level gymnasts. Foot Ankle Spec 2015;8(2):130–4.
4. Kramer DE, Mahan ST, Hresko MT. Displaced intra-articular fractures of the great toe in children: intervene with caution! J Pediatr Orthop 2014;34(2):144–9.
5. Crawford AH, Mehlman CT, Parikh SN. Fractures and dislocations of the foot and ankle. In: Mencio GA, Swiontkowski MF, editors. Green's skeletal trauma in children. 5th edition. Philadelphia: Elsevier Saunders; 2015. p. 473–542.
6. Crawford H. Fractures and dislocations of the foot. In: Flynn JM, Skaggs DL, Waters PM, editors. Rockwood and Wilkins' fracture in children. 8th edition. Philadelphia: Wolters Kluwer; 2015. p. 1225–70.
7. Available at: http://www.cdc.gov/arthritis/basics/risk-factors.htm. Accessed October 6, 2016.
8. Pinckney LE, Currarino G, Kennedy LA. The stubbed great toe: a cause of occult compound fracture and infection. Radiology 1981;138(2):375–7.
9. Reyes BA, Ho CA. The high risk of infection with delayed treatment of open Seymour fractures: Salter-Harris I/II or juxta-epiphyseal fractures of the distal phalanx with associated nailbed laceration. J Pediatr Orthop 2015. [Epub ahead of print].
10. Koval KJ, Zuckerman JD. Pediatric foot. In: Handbook of fractures. 3rd edition. Philadelphia: Wolters Kluwer; 2006. p. 639.
11. Herrera-Soto JA, Scherb M, Duffy MF, et al. Fractures of the fifth metatarsal in children and adolescents. J Pediatr Orthop 2007;27(4):427–31.
12. Myerson MS. Experimental decompression of the fascial compartments of the foot – the basis for fasciotomy in acute compartment syndromes. Foot Ankle 1988;8(6):308–14.
13. Manoli A, Fakhouri A, Weber T. Compartmental catheterization and fasciotomy of the foot. Oper Tech Orthop 1992;2:203–10.
14. Wallin K, Nguyen H, Russell L, et al. Acute traumatic compartment syndrome in pediatric foot: A systematic review and case report. J Foot Ankle Surg 2016;55(4):817–20.

15. Silas SI, Herzenberg JE, Myerson MS, et al. Compartment syndrome of the foot in children. J Bone Joint Surg Am 1995;77(3):356–61.

16. Bibbo C, Lin SS, Cunningham FJ. Acute traumatic compartment syndrome of the foot in children. Pediatr Emerg Care 2000;16(4):244–8.

17. Trevino SG, Kodros S. Controversies in tarsometatarsal injuries. Orthop Clin North Am 1995;26:229–38.

18. Wiley JJ. Tarsometatarsal joint injuries in children. J Pediatr Orthop 1981;1(3):255–60.

19. Buoncristiani AM, Manos RE, Mills WJ. Plantarflexion tarsometatarsal joint injuries in children. J Pediatr Orthop 2001;21(3):324–7.

20. Denning JR, Butler L, Eismann EA, et al. Functional outcomes and health-related quality of life following pediatric Lisfranc tarsometatarsal injury treatment. 2015 May, Pediatric Orthopaedic Society of North America Annual Meeting, paper 159, in press.

21. Englanoff G, Anglin D, Hutson HR. Lisfranc fracture-dislocation: a frequently missed diagnosis in the emergency department. Ann Emerg Med 1995;26: 229–33.

22. Peterson L, Romanus B, Dahlberg E. Fracture of the collum tali—an experimental study. J Biomech 1976;9(4):277–9.

23. Smith JT, Curtis RA, Spencer S, et al. Complications of talus fractures in children. J Pediatr Orthop 2010; 30(8):779–84.

24. Rammelt S, Zwipp H, Gavlik JM. Avascular necrosis after minimally displaced talus fracture in a child. Foot Ankle Int 2000;21(12):1030–6.

25. Hawkins LG. Fractures of the neck of the talus. J Bone Joint Surg Am 1970;52(5):991–1002.

26. Ogden J. The foot. In: Ogden J, editor. Skeletal injury in the child. New York: Springer Verlag; 2000. p. 626–7.

27. Meier R, Krettek C, Griensven M, et al. Fractures of the talus in the pediatric patient. Foot Ankle Surg 2005;11:5–10.

28. Thermann H, Hufner T, Richter M, et al. Paediatric foot fractures. Foot Ankle Surg 2001;7:61–76.

29. Perumal V, Wall E, Babekir N. Juvenile osteochondritis dissecans of the talus. J Pediatr Orthop 2007;27(7):821–5.

30. Canale ST, Belding RH. Osteochondral lesions of the talus. J Bone Joint Surg Am 1980;62(1):97–102.

31. Brunet JA. Calcaneal fractures in children: long-term results of treatment. J Bone Joint Surg Br 2000;82B:211–6.

32. Ribbans WJ, Natarajan R, Alavala S. Pediatric foot fractures. Clin Orthop Relat Res 2005;432:107–15.

33. Feng Y, Yu Y, Shui X, et al. Closed reduction and percutaneous fixation of calcaneus fractures in children. Orthopedics 2016;39(4):e744–8.

34. Schmidt TL, Weiner DS. Calcaneal fractures in children. An evaluation of the nature of the injury in 56 children. Clin Orthop Relat Res 1982;(171): 150–5.

35. Wiley JJ, Profitt A. Fractures of the os calcis in children. Clin Orthop Relat Res 1984;188:131–8.

36. Pickle A, Benaroch TE, Guy P, et al. Clinical outcome of pediatric calcaneal fractures treated with open reduction and internal fixation. J Pediatr Orthop 2004;24(2):178–80.

37. Summers H, Kramer PA, Benirschke SK. Pediatric calcaneal fractures. Orthop Rev 2009;1(e9):30–3.

38. Rapariz JM, Ocete G, Gonzalez-Herranz P, et al. Distal tibial triplane fractures: long-term follow-up. J Pediatr Orthop 1996;16(1):113–8.

39. Karrholm J. The triplane fracture: four years of follow-up of 21 cases and review of the literature. J Pediatr Orthop B 1997;6(2):91–102.

40. Eismann EA, Stephan ZA, Mehlman CT, et al. Pediatric triplane ankle fractures: Impact of radiographs and computed tomography on fracture classification and treatment planning. J Bone Joint Surg Am 2015;97(12):995–1002.

41. Spiegel PG, Cooperman DR, Laros GS. Epiphyseal fractures of the distal ends of the tibia and fibula. A retrospective study of two hundred and thirty-seven cases in children. J Bone Joint Surg Am 1978;60(8):1046–50.

42. De Sanctis N, Della Corte S, Pempinello C. Distal tibial and fibular epiphyseal fractures in children: Prognostic criteria and long-term results in 158 patients. J Pediatr Orthop B 2000;9(1):40–4.

43. Russo F, Moor MA, Mubarak SJ, et al. Salter Harris II fracture of the distal tibia: does surgical management reduce the risk of premature physeal closure? J Pediatr Orthop 2013;33(5):524–9.

44. Seel EH, Noble S, Clarke NM, et al. Outcome of distal tibial physeal injuries. J Pediatr Orthop B 2011;20(4):242–8.

45. Cai H, Wang Z, Cai H. Surgical indications for distal tibial epiphyseal fractures in children. Orthopedics 2015;38(3):e189–95.

46. Rohmiller MT, Gaynor TP, Pawelek J, et al. Salter-Harris I and II fracture of the distal tibia: does mechanism of injury relate to premature physeal closure? J Pediatr Orthop 2006;26(3):322–8.

47. Nenopoulos SP, Papavasiliou VA, Papavasiliou AV. Outcome of physeal and epiphyseal injuries of the distal tibia with intraarticular involvement. J Pediatr Orthop 2005;25(4):518–22.

48. Berson L, Davidson RS, Dormans JP, et al. Growth disturbances after distal tibial physeal fracture. Foot Ankle Int 2000;21(1):54–8.

49. Ecklund K, Jaramillo D. Patterns of premature physeal arrest: MR imaging of 111 children. AJR Am J Roentgenol 2002;178(4):967–72.

50. Herman MJ, Ranade A. Ankle fractures in children. In: McCarthy JJ, Drennan JC, editors. Drennan's the child's foot and ankle. 2nd edition.

Philadelphia: Wolters Kluwer Lippincott Williams & Wilkins; 2010. p. 356–78.

51. Phan VC, Wroten E, Yngve DA. Foot progression angle after distal tibial physeal fracture. J Pediatr Orthop 2002;22(1):31–5.

52. Cooperman DR, Spiegel PG, Laros GS. Tibial fractures involving the ankle in children. The so-called triplane epiphyseal fracture. J Bone Joint Surg Am 1978;60(8):1040–6.

53. Crawford AH. Ankle fractures in children. Instr Course Lect 1995;44:317–24.

54. Healy WA 3rd, Starkweather KD, Meyer J, et al. Triplane fractures associated with proximal third fibula fracture. Am J Orthop 1996;25:449–51.

55. Mubarak SJ. Extensor retinaculum syndrome of the ankle after injury to the distal tibial physis. J Bone Joint Surg Br 2002;84B(1):11–4.

56. Wilder RT. Management of pediatric patients with complex regional pain syndrome. Clin J Pain 2006;22(5):443–8.

57. Sarrail R, Launay F, Marez M. Reflex dystrophy in children and adolescents. J Bone Joint Surg Br 2004;86(Suppl):23.

58. Dietz FR, Mathews KD, Montgomery WJ. Reflex sympathetic dystrophy in children. Clin Orthop Relat Res 1990;258:225–31.

59. Wilder RT, Berde CB, Wolohan M, et al. Reflex sympathetic dystrophy in children. Clinical characteristics and follow-up of 70 patients. J Bone Joint Surg Am 1992;74(6):910–9.

60. Dietz FR, Compton SP. Outcomes of simple treatment for complex regional pain syndrome type I in children. Iowa Orthop J 2015;35:175–80.

61. Tan EC, van de Sandt-Renkema N, Krabbe PF, et al. Quality of life in adults with childhood-onset of complex regional pain syndrome type I. Injury 2009;40(8):901–4.

62. Caterini R, Farsetti P, Ippolito E. Long-term followup of physeal injury to the ankle. Foot Ankle 1991;11(6):372–83.

63. Ertl JP, Barrach RL, Alexander AH, et al. Triplane fracture of the distal tibial epiphysis. Long-term follow-up. J Bone Joint Surg Am 1988;70(7):967–76.

64. Tarr RR, Resnick CT, Wagner KS, et al. Changes in tibiotalar joint contact areas following experimentally induced tibial angular deformities. Clin Orthop Relat Res 1985;199:72–80.

65. Murphy RF, Naqvi M, Miller PE, et al. Pediatric orthopaedic lower extremity trauma and venous thromboembolism. J Child Orthop 2015;9(5):381–4.

66. Ceroni D, Martin X, Delhumeau C, et al. Effects of cast-mediated immobilization on bone mineral mass at various sites in adolescents with lower-extremity fracture. J Bone Joint Surg Am 2012;94(3):208–11.

Upper Extremity

Controversies in Fractures of the Proximal Ulna

Christopher M. Hopkins, MD, James H. Calandruccio, MD, Benjamin M. Mauck, MD*

KEYWORDS

- Proximal ulna • Fracture • Olecranon process • Coronoid process • Treatment

KEY POINTS

- The olecranon and coronoid processes are important components of the complex proximal ulna, providing bony stability and attachment sites for many important muscles and ligaments.
- Most olecranon fractures are best treated operatively with tension-band wiring or plate fixation; plate fixation appears to be preferable for comminuted fractures.
- Some isolated displaced (>2 mm) olecranon fractures in elderly patients can be successfully treated nonoperatively.
- Coronoid fractures generally should be treated operatively, regardless of size, if there is associated instability; both the "lasso" technique and the suture anchors have produced good outcomes.
- Anteromedial facet fractures deserve special attention because of the facet's contribution to elbow stability; most fractures require rigid fixation unless small and clinical examination demonstrates elbow stability.

ANATOMIC CONSIDERATIONS

The anatomy of the proximal ulna is complex, and restoration of anatomic alignment is essential to restore normal biomechanics and avoid early arthritis, subluxation, and loss of function. Several studies have described anatomic features of the ulna that must be restored. Recently, much has been published on the proximal ulna dorsal angulation (PUDA) (Fig. 1). Rouleau and colleagues[1–3] characterized the PUDA in 50 patients examining bilateral elbow radiographs. They found a PUDA to be present in 96% of study participants with an average PUDA of 5.7° (range, 0–14). The average tip to apex distance was 47 mm (range, 34–78 mm). Both measurements were found to have good intrareliability and interreliability.

IMAGING

Historically, imaging evaluation of proximal ulnar fractures has consisted of a standard anteroposterior and lateral elbow series supplemented with a radiocapitellar view as needed[4] (Fig. 2). However, recent improvements in imaging techniques and availability of 3-dimensional (3D) computed tomographic (CT) reconstructions have led some investigators to recommend more advanced imaging in certain fracture patterns.[1] In their retrospective review evaluating the use of 2.7-mm and 2.4-mm plates, Wellman and colleagues[5] found that 6 of 7 fractures thought to be a simple pattern on preoperative radiographs had occult comminution on CT scan. These investigators cautioned against using tension-band wiring (TBW) for fixation because many fractures may displace because of comminution not seen on standard plain films.

OLECRANON FRACTURES

Nonoperative Management

Olecranon fractures generally are managed operatively; however, nonoperative management is

---

Disclosures: The authors have no conflicts to disclose.
Department of Orthopaedic Surgery and Biomedical Engineering, University of Tennessee–Campbell Clinic, 1211 Union Avenue, Suite 510, Memphis, TN 38104, USA
* Corresponding author. 1211 Union Avenue, Suite 510, Memphis, TN 38104.
E-mail address: bmauck31@gmail.com

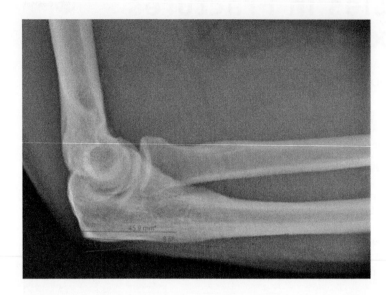

Fig. 1. PUDA measurement and tip-to-apex distance.

indicated in select cases. Conventional teaching has recommended that fractures with less than 2 mm of articular displacement and with an intact extensor mechanism should be treated nonoperatively.[4] Duckworth and colleagues[6] reported encouraging results with nonoperative treatment of isolated displaced (>2 mm) olecranon fractures in elderly patients. In their series of 43 patients with a mean age of 76 years, 72% had good to excellent results at 4 months, a Disabilities of the Arm, Shoulder, and Hand (DASH) score of 2.9, and an Oxford elbow score of 47, with a 91% satisfaction at 6 years. Veras del Monte and colleagues[7] also reported good results after nonoperative treatment of displaced olecranon fractures in 12 elderly (mean age 82 years) patients. At final follow-up (average 15 months), no patient had any limitation in activity of daily living, and 8 of the 12 were asymptomatic with acceptable ranges of motion (ROMs). Clinical results were good in 8, fair in 3, and poor in one

despite 9 fibrous nonunions. Eleven of the 12 patients graded their treatment as excellent.

Excision and Triceps Advancement

Olecranon excision with triceps advancement has been advocated as a viable treatment option in elderly patients with a comminuted fracture proximal to the coronoid with intact medial collateral ligament, distal radioulnar joint, and intraosseous membrane.[8,9] The indications, technique for triceps attachment, and amount of olecranon that can be excised remain controversial. In the largest study to date, Gartsman and colleagues[10] compared 53 isolated displaced olecranon fractures treated with primary excision to 54 treated with open reduction and internal fixation (ORIF). The groups had similar motion, function, pain, elbow stability, and incidence of posttraumatic arthritis; however, the complication rate was much higher in the ORIF group (23% compared with 4% in the excision

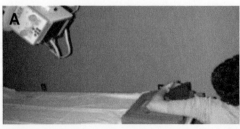
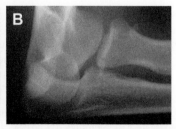

Fig. 2. (A) Positioning and (B) radiographic appearance of the radiocapitellar view. Obtained with elbow positioned for lateral radiograph but with radiograph beam angled 45° cephalad. (From King GJW. Fractures of the head of the radius. In: Wolfe S, Pederson W, Hotchkiss R, et al, editors. Green's operative hand surgery. 6th edition. Philadelphia: Elsevier; 2011. p. 784; with permission.)

group). In addition, biomechanical testing showed no difference in elbow extension between groups.

The amount of olecranon that can be removed before instability occurs has been debated. McKeever and Buck[11] stated that as much as 80% could be excised without compromising elbow stability; however, Bell and colleagues[12,13] performed serial resections and triceps advancements on 8 cadaver specimens and determined elbow stability after various amounts of olecranon resection. They noted instability to varus-valgus angulation and ulnohumeral rotation after resection of as little as 12.5%, with a progressive increase in instability up to 75%. Gross instability was noted after resection of 87.5%. Gartsman and colleagues[10] found that one of their 54 patients treated with excision developed instability when 75% of the olecranon was excised. An and colleagues[14] evaluated elbow stability after varying amounts of proximal ulnar resection and found a linear decrease in elbow constraint with increasing amounts of resection. They concluded that with resection of more than 50%, instability may occur; however, Inhofe and Howard[15] reported that 11 of 12 patients had good or excellent results after excision of as much as 70%.

Tension Band Wiring or Plate Fixation

Before the advent of contoured proximal ulnar plates, displaced olecranon fractures were traditionally managed with TBW. This technique, in which tensile forces from the triceps are converted to compressive forces at the articular surface, has been advocated by the Arbeitsgemeinschaft für Osteosynthesefragen group.[16] Long-standing debate exists regarding the method of TBW and indications for its use. In recent years, fixation using one-third tubular, dynamic compression, pelvic reconstruction, and, most recently, anatomically precontoured plate fixation has been advocated.

TBW is most often recommended for simple, transverse olecranon fractures without distal extension.[17] The TBW construct consists of 2 longitudinal Kirschner wires and a wire placed in a figure-of-8 fashion through the dorsal cortex distal to the fracture and looped over the bent ends of the Kirschner wires proximally that are buried under the triceps (Fig. 3). The proper location of the Kirschner wires has been recommended to be in the anterior cortex for bicortical fixation; however, concern over damage to neurovascular structures and penetration of the proximal radioulnar joint has led some investigators to advocate fixation in the distal or proximal

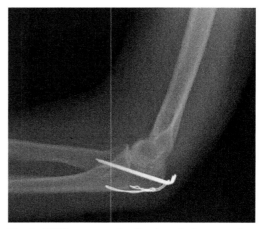

Fig. 3. TBW construct for fixation of olecranon fracture. (Reprinted with permission from Amini MH, Azar FM, Wilson BR, et al. Comparison of outcomes and costs of tension-band and locking-plate osteosynthesis in transverse olecranon fractures: a matched-cohort study. Am J Orthop (Belle Mead NJ) 2015;44:E211. Copyright The American Journal of Orthopedics. All rights reserved.)

ulnar canal. Huang and colleagues[18] reviewed 78 displaced olecranon fractures treated with TBW fixation with 3 different Kirschner wire placement techniques: proximal ulnar canal, anterior ulnar cortex, and distal ulnar canal. They found proximal pin migration and elbow irritation when the wires were placed in the proximal ulnar canal and advocated placement in the distal canal to obtain adequate purchase and avoid the risk associated with anterior cortical penetration.[19–22] In addition, in a review of 62 patients by Chalidis and colleagues,[23] there was no difference in pin loosening or back-out whether or not the anterior cortex was engaged.

The use of TBW in comminuted fractures is debatable. Hume and Wiss[19] compared fixation with a one-third tubular plate to fixation with TBW in 41 patients with displaced olecranon fractures. Plate fixation took on average 25 minutes longer, but the frequency of symptomatic hardware was much higher in the TBW group (42% vs 5%), as was loss of reduction resulting in significant articular step-off (>2 mm) (53% vs 5%). Clinical and radiographic results also were better in the group with plate fixation.[19] Cadaver studies have shown plate fixation to be more stable than TBW in a comminuted fracture model.[24] The recent advent of anatomic locked precontoured plates has led some investigators to recommend locked plate fixation for fractures with distal extension, dorsal comminution, or a high-energy mechanism. Lan and colleagues[25] compared the outcomes in 10 patients treated with nonlocked plating to those in 14 patients treated with anatomic locked plating and found no difference in Mayo Elbow Performance Index (MEPI), ROM, and patient satisfaction. Schliemann and colleagues[26] compared TBW to locking compression plate fixation in displaced, noncomminuted olecranon fractures. With 13 patients in each group, at an average follow-up of 43 months, the investigators found more good to excellent results based on mayo elbow performance score (92% vs 77%) and less frequent need for hardware removal (7 vs 12) in the plate group, but radiographic and clinical outcomes were similar. They concluded that given the higher overall cost of locked plate fixation, TBW was the treatment of choice for Mayo IIA olecranon fractures (Fig. 4). However, given the small number of patients in the study, it is possible that it was underpowered to show a clinical difference. Moreover, no cost analysis was performed to examine the additional cost of hardware removal. The rate of hardware removal following TBW or plate fixation has varied considerably in the literature, ranging from 11% to 80% for TBW[22,27–29] and 0% to 51% for plate fixation.[5,19,30,31] Anderson and colleagues[32] reported on the use of the Mayo Congruent Elbow Plate System for displaced olecranon fractures and found that only 3 of 32 patients required hardware removal.

CORONOID FRACTURES

The coronoid is important to the ulnohumeral joint stability. Along with the radial head, it provides resistance to posterior displacement of the ulna on the distal humerus. In addition, the anteromedial facet provides stability against varus force.[33] Along with its bony contribution to stability of the elbow, the coronoid also serves to stabilize the elbow joint through its insertion of the brachialis muscle, the anterior joint capsule, and the medial ulnar collateral ligament. Much has been published regarding the classification, diagnosis, and management of these often complex injuries, but there is still no clear consensus.

Anatomy/Classification
Classification of coronoid fractures has typically been based on size using the Regan and Morrey classification.[34] Many investigators contend that

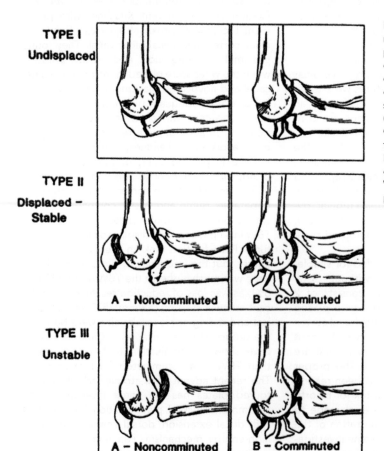

Fig. 4. Mayo classification of olecranon fractures. Type I, nondisplaced, noncomminuted (IA) or comminuted (IB). Type II, stable, displaced, noncomminuted (IIA) or comminuted (IIB). Type III, unstable, displaced, noncomminuted (IIIA) or comminuted (IIIB). (*From* Cabenela ME, Morrey BF. Fractures of the olecranon. In: Morrey BF, editor. The elbow and its disorders. 3rd edition. Philadelphia: WB Saunders/Elsevier; 2000; with permission.)

TYPE I
Undisplaced

TYPE II
Displaced –
Stable

A – Noncomminuted   B – Comminuted

TYPE III
Unstable

A – Noncomminuted   B – Comminuted

the O'Driscoll classification, which is based on a fracture pattern that is associated with the overall pattern of injury, is more helpful to guide treatment.[35] Doornberg and Ring[36] examined 67 coronoid fractures and was able to confirm a strong association between O'Driscoll fracture type and mechanism of injury. The pattern of injury was classified as an olecranon fracture-dislocation (anterior or posterior), terrible triad, or varus posteromedial rotational instability pattern. They showed that olecranon fracture-dislocations were associated with large (>50%) coronoid fractures in 22 of 24 patients, whereas 31 of 32 terrible triad patterns had associated small (<50%) coronoid fractures. Of the 11 patients in the varus posteromedial instability group, all had fractures of the anteromedial facet.[36] However, there has been little published on how to properly measure the coronoid height. Matzon and colleagues[37] used 35 cadaver arms and a 3D digitizing system to define coronoid anatomy. Their results suggest that coronoid height is best defined by the trough of the trochlear notch and the slope change of the distal coronoid process (Fig. 5).

Coronoid fractures associated with "terrible triad" injuries are approached through either a lateral approach (Kaplan or Kocher) or a posterior approach. Coronoid fractures involving the anteromedial facet are better exposed from a medial approach; however, debate remains as to whether a flexor carpi ulnaris (FCU)-split or Hotchkiss over-the-top approach provides better exposure. Huh and colleagues[38] examined 20 cadavers and using imaging software concluded that the FCU-split approach (Fig. 6) provided 3 times greater surface area exposure and that the Hotchkiss approach (Fig. 7) failed to expose the sublime tubercle and posterior bundle of medial collateral ligament (MCL) in most cadavers.

Imaging

Coronoid fractures have been traditionally assessed on a lateral radiograph of the elbow,[34] but, because the fracture often is small and can be difficult to adequately evaluate when there are concomitant fractures, CT scanning has been recommended to further delineate the size and location of the coronoid fracture.[39–43] Adams and colleagues[44] sought to determine the reliability of CT (with 3D reconstruction) in assessing coronoid fracture patterns using the Regan-Morrey classification system (Fig. 8). With 3 reviewers examining 52 CT scans, they reported good to very good interobserver and intraobserver reliability. Lindenhovius and colleagues[45] examined the intraobserver and interobserver reliability of 2D versus 3D CT scanning in assessing fracture characteristics and classifying coronoid fractures. Twenty-nine orthopedic surgeons examined 10 fractures. The investigators found better interobserver reliability with both the Regan and Morrey and the O'Driscoll classifications using 3D CT scans. More recently, Mellema and colleagues[46] recommended the use of quantitative 3D CT to quantify fracture fragment volume, number of fracture fragments, and level of articular surface involvement. They found significant variability when looking at fracture types and injury patterns and suggested that quantitative 3D CT may aid in preoperative planning.

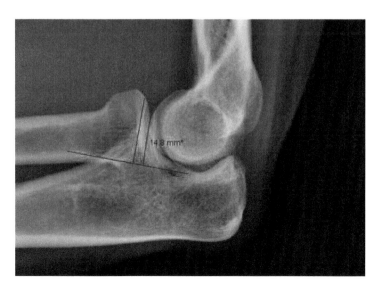

Fig. 5. Measurement of coronoid height. (*Data from* Matzon JL, Widmer BJ, Draganich LF, et al. Anatomy of the coronoid process. J Hand Surg Am 2006;31(8):1272–8.)

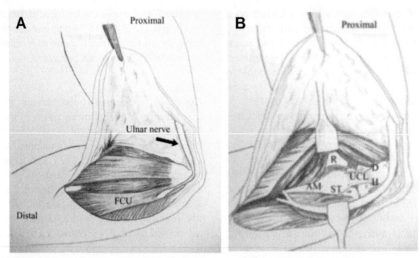

Fig. 6. FCU-split approach showing initial (*A*) and deep (*B*) exposure. AM, anteromedial facet; DH, distal humerus; R, radial head; ST, sublime tubercle. (*From* Huh J, Krueger CA, Medvecky MJ, et al. Skeletal Trauma Research Consortium (STReC). Medial elbow exposure for coronoid fractures: FCU-split versus over-the-top. J Orthop Trauma 2013;27:731; with permission.)

Nonoperative Management

Most investigators recommend treating coronoid fractures operatively, regardless of size, if there is associated instability[47–50] because unsatisfactory results have been reported after nonoperative treatment of coronoid fractures.[50,51] However, Jeon and colleagues[52] demonstrated in a cadaver study that Regan and Morrey types I and II coronoid fractures did not affect elbow stability with an intact radial head and lateral ligament

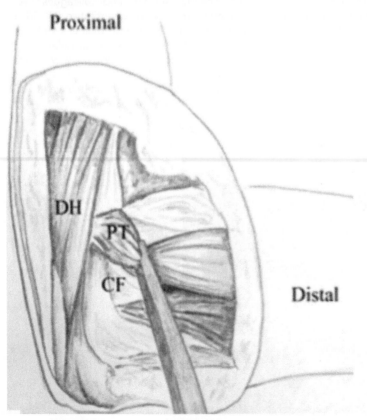

Fig. 7. Hotchkiss over-the-top approach. CF, common flexor origin; PT, pronator teres. (*From* Huh J, Krueger CA, Medvecky MJ, et al. Skeletal Trauma Research Consortium (STReC). Medial elbow exposure for coronoid fractures: FCU-split versus over-the-top. J Orthop Trauma 2013;27:732; with permission.)

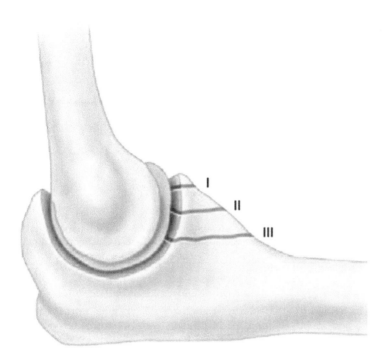

Fig. 8. Regan and Morrey classification of the coronoid based on degree of involvement. (*From* Perez EA. Fractures of the shoulder, arm, and forearm. In: Canale ST, Beaty JH, editors. Campbell's operative orthopaedics. 12th edition. Philadelphia: Elsevier; 2013. p. 2872; with permission.)

complex. Papatheodorou and colleagues[53] expanded on this concept in a clinical study in which they reviewed the outcomes of 14 consecutive patients with Regan and Morrey type I (2 patients) or type II (12 patients) fractures treated nonoperatively. All patients had radial head repair or reconstruction and repair of the lateral ulnar collateral ligament (LUCL). They reported a mean arc of motion of 123°, mean Bromberg and Morrey score of 90, and DASH score of 14 at an average of 24 months.

Chan and colleagues[54,55] described 11 patients with terrible triad injuries and Regan-Morrey type I or II fractures managed nonoperatively. Inclusion criteria were a concentric joint reduction, radial head fracture without mechanical block to rotation, small coronoid fracture, and stable arc of motion to a minimum of 30° of extension. At a minimum 1-year follow-up, the mean DASH score was 8, mean MEPI was 94, mean ROM was 135°, and no instability was reported. One patient required surgical stabilization for recurrent instability. The investigators concluded that nonoperative treatment of coronoid fractures is appropriate in carefully selected patients with close follow-up.

Methods of Fixation

Proposed techniques described for coronoid fracture fixation include screw, plate, Kirschner wire, suture anchor, and suture techniques.[35,36,50,56] In

an attempt to clarify the best fixation technique, Garrigues and colleagues[47] retrospectively reviewed 40 consecutive patients with Regan and Morrey type I and II fractures with a minimum of 18 months of follow-up. They compared

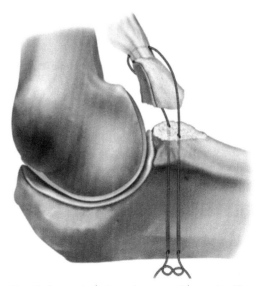

Fig. 9. Lasso technique in coronoid repair. (*From* Garrigues GE, Wray WH III, Lindenhovius ALC, et al. Fixation of the coronoid process in elbow fracture-dislocations. J Bone Joint Surg Am 2011;93:1876; with permission.)

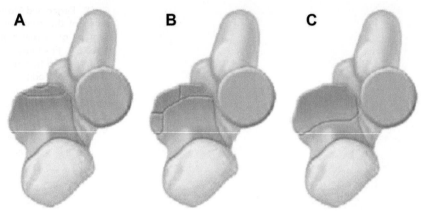

Fig. 10. O'Driscoll classification of coronoid fractures based on fragmentation pattern. (*A*) Type I, transverse tip fracture. (*B*) Type II, fracture of the anteromedial facet. (*C*) Type III, fracture through the base. (*From* Perez EA. Fractures of the shoulder, arm, and forearm. In: Canale ST, Beaty JH, editors. Campbell's operative orthopaedics. 12th edition. Philadelphia: Elsevier; 2013. p. 2872; with permission.)

the "lasso" technique (28 patients) to ORIF with screw or suture anchor (12 patients) and found that the lasso technique (Fig. 9) was more stable both intraoperatively and at final follow-up, with a lower frequency of implant failure resulting in malunion and nonunion. Clarke and colleagues[57] retrospectively reviewed 3 patients with terrible triad injuries and type 1 coronoid fractures and found that the use of suture anchor fixation produced outcomes comparable to those reported in the literature. They concluded that suture anchors offer a simpler, quicker method of coronoid fixation with adequate fixation.

Anteromedial Facet Fracture

Recently, coronoid fractures involving the anteromedial facet (O'Driscoll type II) have received attention because of their associated injuries and potentially poor results when managed conservatively.[35,36] These fractures are classified into 3 types based on the amount of the anteromedial facet involved. Type I involves a rim fracture; type II, a rim and tip; and type III, the rim and sublime tubercle with or without the tip (Fig. 10).[35]

Although the general recommendation has been to fix all anteromedial facet fractures, Chan and colleagues[54] reported nonoperative treatment of 9 type II fractures and one type III fracture. At a mean follow-up of 50 months, ROM was 2° to 137°, mean patient-rated elbow evaluation score was 9, MEPI score was 94, and DASH was 7 with no evidence of recurrent instability. They recommended consideration of nonoperative management for fractures that are small and minimally displaced with no evidence of elbow subluxation. The optimal operative management of anteromedial facet

fractures is controversial. In their retrospective series of 11 patients with isolated anteromedial facet fractures, Park and colleagues[58] described their protocol involving repair of the LUCL only in type I fractures and buttress plating and LUCL repair in types II and III. Their results were encouraging, with an average ROM of 128° and average MEPI of 89.

SUMMARY

Treatment of proximal ulnar fractures continues to evolve as the understanding of these complex injuries and the implants available to manage them continues to improve. Optimal management of olecranon fractures depends on multiple patient-related and surgeon-related factors. The literature has shown favorable outcomes with nonoperative management of displaced olecranon fracture in properly selected patients. The management of displaced olecranon fractures in younger patients continues to be debated between TBW and various plate options, with most recent studies recommending plate fixation for comminuted fracture patterns.

Coronoid fracture management has continued to change, with a trend toward more aggressive management as the understanding of the anatomy and function improves. Imaging modalities with 3D CT allow more complete evaluation and classification of fractures. Although most coronoid fractures require operative intervention, some coronoid fractures demonstrate enough stability to be managed without surgery. When operative fixation is necessary, coronoid fractures can be fixed with either a lasso technique or suture anchors when small or screw fixation, with or without buttress plating, when large. Management of anteromedial facet fractures deserves special attention given its contribution to elbow stability. Most fractures require rigid fixation unless small, and clinical examination demonstrates elbow stability.

REFERENCES

1. Rouleau DM, Sandman E, van Riet R, et al. Management of fractures of the proximal ulna. J Am Acad Orthop Surg 2013;21:149–60.
2. Storen G. Traumatic dislocation of the radial head as an isolated lesion in children; report of one case with special regard to roentgen diagnosis. Acta Chir Scand 1959;116:144–7.
3. Rouleau DM, Sandman E, Canet F, et al. Radial head translation measurement in healthy individuals: the radiocapitellar ratio. J Shoulder Elbow Surg 2012;21:574–9.
4. Ring D. Elbow fractures and dislocations. In: Bucholz RW, Court-Brown CM, Heckman JD, et al, editors. Rockwood and Green's fractures in adults. 7th edition. Philadelphia: Lippincott Williams & Wilkins; 2010. p. 905–44.
5. Wellman DS, Lazaro LE, Cymerman RM, et al. Treatment of olecranon fractures with 2.4- and 2.7-mm plating techniques. J Orthop Trauma 2015;29:36–43.
6. Duckworth AD, Bugler KE, Clement ND, et al. Nonoperative management of displaced olecranon fractures in low-demand elderly patients. J Bone Joint Surg Am 2014;96:67–72.
7. Veras Del Monte L, Sirera Vercher M, Busquets Net R, et al. Conservative treatment of displaced fractures of the olecranon in the elderly. Injury 1999;30:105–10.
8. Teasdall R, Savoie FH, Hughes JL. Comminuted fractures of the proximal radius and ulna. Clin Orthop Relat Res 1993;292:37–47.
9. Hak DJ, Golladay GJ. Olecranon fractures: treatment options. J Am Acad Orthop Surg 2000;8:266–75.
10. Gartsman GM, Sculco TP, Otis JC. Operative treatment of olecranon fractures: excision or open reduction with internal fixation. J Bone Joint Surg Am 1981;63:718–21.
11. McKeever FM, Buck RM. Fracture of the olecranon process of the ulna: treatment by excision of fragment and repair of triceps tendon. JAMA 1947;135:1–5.
12. Bell TH, Ferreira LM, McDonald CP, et al. Contribution of the olecranon to elbow stability: an in vitro biomechanical study. J Bone Joint Surg Am 2010;92:949–57.
13. Wilson J, Bajwa A, Kamath V, et al. Biomechanical comparison of interfragmentary compression in transverse fractures of the olecranon. J Bone Joint Surg Br 2011;93:245–50.
14. An KN, Morrey BF, Chao EY. The effect of partial removal of proximal ulna on elbow constraint. Clin Orthop Relat Res 1986;(209):270–9.
15. Inhofe PD, Howard TC. The treatment of olecranon fractures by excision or fragments and repair of the extensor mechanism: historical review and report of 12 fractures. Orthopedics 1993;16:1313–7.
16. Morrey BF. Current concepts in the treatment of fractures of the radial head, the olecranon, and the coronoid. J Bone Joint Surg Am 1995;77:316–27.
17. Schatzker J. Fractures of the olecranon. In: Schatzker J, Tile M, editors. The rationale of operative fracture care. Berlin: Springer-Verlag; 1987. p. 89–95.
18. Huang TW, Wu CC, Fan KF, et al. Tension band wiring for olecranon fractures: relative stability of Kirschner wires in various configurations. J Trauma 2010;68:173–6.
19. Hume MC, Wiss DA. Olecranon fractures. A clinical and radiographic comparison of tension band wiring and plate fixation. Clin Orthop Relat Res 1992;(285):229–35.
20. Hotchkiss RN. Fractures of the olecranon. In: Rockwood CA Jr, Green DP, Bucholz RW, et al, editors. Rockwood and Green's fractures in adults. 4th edition. Philadelphia: JB Lippincott; 1996. p. 984–96.
21. Rettig AC, Waugh TR, Evanski PM. Fracture of the olecranon: a problem of management. J Trauma 1979;19:23–8.
22. Wolfgang G, Burke F, Bush D, et al. Surgical treatment of displaced olecranon fractures by tension band wiring technique. Clin Orthop Relat Res 1987;(224):192–204.
23. Chalidis BE, Sachinis NC, Samoladas EP, et al. Is tension band wiring technique the "gold standard" for the treatment of olecranon fractures? A long term functional outcome study. J Orthop Surg Res 2008;3:9.
24. Fyfe IS, Mossad MM, Holdsworth BJ. Methods of fixation of olecranon fractures. An experimental mechanical study. J Bone Joint Surg Br 1985;67:367–72.
25. Lan TY, Chen CY, Liao PF, et al. Comminuted olecranon fractures treated with anatomically preshaped locking and nonlocking plates: a retrospective comparative study. Formosan Journal of Musculoskeletal Disorders 2013;4:1–5.
26. Schliemann B, Raschke MJ, Groene P, et al. Comparison of tension band wiring and precontoured locking compression plate fixation in Mayo type IIA olecranon fractures. Acta Orthop Belg 2014;80:106–11.
27. Macko D, Szabo RM. Complications of tension-band wiring of olecranon fractures. J Bone Joint Surg Am 1985;67:1396–401.

28. Karlsson MK, Hasserius R, Karlsson C, et al. Fractures of the olecranon: a 15- to 25-year followup of 73 patients. Clin Orthop Relat Res 2002;(403):205–12.

29. Murphy DF, Greene WB, Dameron TB Jr. Displaced olecranon fractures in adults. Clinical evaluation. Clin Orthop Relat Res 1987;(224):215–23.

30. Bailey CS, MacDermid J, Patterson SD, et al. Outcome of plate fixation of olecranon fractures. J Orthop Trauma 2001;15:542–8.

31. Tejwani NC, Garnham IR, Wolinsky PR, et al. Posterior olecranon plating: biomechanical and clinical evaluation of a new operative technique. Bull Hosp Jt Dis 2002;61:27–31.

32. Anderson ML, Larson AN, Merten SM, et al. Congruent elbow plate fixation of olecranon fractures. J Orthop Trauma 2007;21:386–93.

33. Steinmann SP. Coronoid process fracture. J Am Acad Orthop Surg 2008;16(9):519–29.

34. Regan W, Morrey B. Fractures of the coronoid process of the ulna. J Bone Joint Surg Am 1989;71: 1348–54.

35. O'Driscoll SW, Jupiter JB, Cohen MS, et al. Difficult elbow fractures: pearls and pitfalls. Instr Course Lect 2003;52:113–34.

36. Doornberg JN, Ring D. Coronoid fracture patterns. J Hand Surg 2006;31:45–52.

37. Matzon JL, Widmer BJ, Draganich LF, et al. Anatomy of the coronoid process. J Hand Surg Am 2006;31(8):1272–8.

38. Huh J, Krueger CA, Medvecky MJ, et al. Medial elbow exposure for coronoid fractures: FCU-split versus over-the-top. J Orthop Trauma 2013;27:730–4.

39. Steinmann SP. Coronoid process fracture. J Am Acad Orthop Surg 2008;16:519–29.

40. Wells J, Ablove RH. Coronoid fractures of the elbow. Clin Med Res 2008;6:40–4.

41. Ring D. Fractures of the coronoid process of the ulna. J Hand Surg Am 2006;31:1679–89.

42. Moon JG, Zobitz ME, An KN, et al. Optimal screw orientation for fixation of coronoid fractures. J Orthop Trauma 2009;23:277–80.

43. Budoff JE, Meyers DN, Ambrose CG. The comparative stability of screw versus plate versus screw and plate coronoid fixation. J Hand Surg Am 2011;36:238–45.

44. Adams JE, Sanchez-Sotelo J, Kallina CF 4th, et al. Fractures of the coronoid: morphology based upon computer tomography scanning. J Shoulder Elbow Surg 2012;21:782–8.

45. Lindenhovius A, Karanicolas PJ, Bhandari M, et al. Interobserver reliability of coronoid fracture classification: two-dimensional versus three-dimensional computed tomography. J Hand Surg 2009;34:1640–6.

46. Mellema JJ, Janssen SJ, Guitton TG, et al. Quantitative 3-dimensional computed tomography measurements of coronoid fractures. J Hand Surg Am 2015;40:526–33.

47. Garrigues GE, Wray WH 3rd, Lindenhovius AL, et al. Fixation of the coronoid process in elbow fracture-dislocations. J Bone Joint Surg Am 2011; 93:1873–81.

48. Mathew PK, Athwal GS, King GJ. Terrible triad injury of the elbow: current concepts. J Am Acad Orthop Surg 2009;17:137–51.

49. Pugh DM, Wild LM, Schemitsch EH, et al. Standard surgical protocol to treat elbow dislocations with radial head and coronoid fractures. J Bone Joint Surg Am 2004;86-A:1122–30.

50. Ring D, Jupiter JB, Zilberfarb J. Posterior dislocation of the elbow with fractures of the radial head and coronoid. J Bone Joint Surg Am 2002;84: 547–51.

51. Josefsson PO, Gentz CF, Johnell O, et al. Dislocations of the elbow and intraarticular fractures. Clin Orthop Relat Res 1989;(246):126–30.

52. Jeon IH, Sanchez-Sotelo J, Zhao K, et al. The contribution of the coronoid and radial head to the stability of the elbow. J Bone Joint Surg Br 2012;94: 86–92.

53. Papatheodorou LK, Rubright JH, Heim KA, et al. Terrible triad injuries of the elbow: does the coronoid always need to be fixed? Clin Orthop Relat Res 2014;472(7):2084–91.

54. Chan K, Faber KJ, King J, et al. Selected anteromedial coronoid fractures can be treated nonoperatively. J Shoulder Elbow Surg 2016;25:1251–7.

55. Chan K, MacDermid JC, Faber KJ, et al. Can we treat select terrible triad injuries nonoperatively? Clin Orthop Relat Res 2014;472:2092–9.

56. McKee MD, Pugh DM, Wild LM, et al. Standard surgical protocol to treat elbow dislocations with radial head and coronoid fractures. Surgical technique. J Bone Joint Surg Am 2005;87(Suppl 1 Pt 1):22–32.

57. Clarke SE, Lee SY, Raphael JR. Coronoid fixation using suture anchors. Hand (N Y) 2009;4:156–60.

58. Park SM, Lee JS, Jung JY, et al. How should anteromedial coronoid facet fracture be managed? A surgical strategy based on O'Driscoll classification and ligament injury. J Shoulder Elbow Surg 2015;24: 74–82.

Foot and Ankle

Posterior Malleolus Fractures

Shay Tenenbaum, MD[a],*, Nachshon Shazar, MD[a], Nathan Bruck, MD[a],
Jason Bariteau, MD[b]

KEYWORDS

- Posterior malleolar fractures • Posterolateral surgical approach • Syndesmotic stability
- Ankle fracture

KEY POINTS

- Posterior malleolus fractures are varied in morphology.
- Posterior malleolar fractures may challenge syndesmotic stability by adversely affecting the functional integrity of posterior syndesmotic ligaments.
- A preoperative computed tomography scan is imperative for the evaluation of fragment size, comminution, articular impaction, and syndesmotic disruption.
- Fragment size (in terms of percentage of articular surface) should not dictate treatment.
- Treatment should restore ankle joint structural integrity by achieving articular congruity, correcting posterior talar translation, addressing articular impaction, removing osteochondral debris, and establishing syndesmotic stability.

INTRODUCTION

Ankle fractures are common, often require surgery, and represent about one-tenth of all fractures.[1] Population based studies have shown that the incidence of ankle fractures has increased significantly since the 1960s, especially for elderly patients.[1–4]

Overall, about two-thirds of ankle fractures are isolated malleolar fractures, one-fourth are bimalleolar, and the remaining 7% are trimalleolar fractures.[1] These incidences are in accordance with a study by Koval and colleagues,[5] although the investigators found that trimalleolar fractures represented about 14% of fractures. Isolated posterior malleolar fractures (PMFs) are rare, with an estimated incidence of about 0.5% to 1% of fractures.[5–7]

An understanding of the posterior malleolus anatomy, the ligamentous attachments, and its contribution to ankle congruity and stability is critical in determining the appropriate treatment. Although management of lateral and medial malleolar fractures is well established, the treatment PMFs, which are heterogeneous in morphology, remains controversial. No consensus exists regarding their recommended management.[8–11]

Anatomy

The ankle joint is a complex, 3-bone joint consisting of the tibial plafond, the distal fibula, and the talus. The ankle joint is saddle-shaped and derives its stability from a combination of bony and ligamentous structures. The significant role of the medial and lateral ligament complexes in ankle congruity and stabilization is well described.[12–16]

In 1932, Henderson[17] described the posterior malleolus as "the anatomic prominence formed by the posterior inferior margin of the articulating surface of the tibia." With regard to PMFs, understanding of the distal tibiofibular joint is crucial in

---

Disclosures: The authors declare no potential conflicts of interest with respect to the research, authorship, and publication of this article. The authors received no financial support.
[a] Department of Orthopedic Surgery, Chaim Sheba Medical Center Hospital at Tel Hashomer, Affiliated to the Sackler Faculty of Medicine, Tel Aviv University, 1 Emek HaEla St, Ramat Gan 52621, Israel; [b] Department of Orthopaedics, Emory University School of Medicine, 59 Executive Park South, Suite 2000, Atlanta, GA 30306, USA
* Corresponding author.
E-mail address: shaytmd@gmail.com

order to formulate appropriate treatment strategies. The distal tibia and fibula form the osseous part of the syndesmosis and are attached by the anterior inferior tibiofibular ligament (AITFL), the posterior inferior tibiofibular ligament (PITFL), the transverse ligament, and the interosseous ligament (IOL).[18] Based on a cadaveric study, Ogilvie-Harris and colleagues[19] showed that 42% of syndesmotic stability is provided by the PITFL, 35% by the AITFL, and 22% by the IOL. Because the PITFL extends from the posterior malleolus to the posterior tubercle of the fibula, PMFs challenge the structural integrity of the posterior syndesmotic ligaments, and may produce syndesmotic disruption (Fig. 1).

Biomechanics

The complex geometry of the tibiotalar joint and its interrelations with static and dynamic stabilizers all influence load characteristics.[20–22] The effects of PMF on ankle joint biomechanics, in terms of stability[23–26] and contact stresses,[20,27–29] have been the subjects of several studies.

Scheidt and colleagues[23] created PMFs involving 25% of the articular surface. The investigators showed that this might lead to excessive internal rotation and posterior instability in a loaded ankle joint. Note that fracture fixation increased ankle stability, but not significantly.

In contrast, other investigators showed no such effect of PMFs on ankle joint stability.

Raasch and colleagues[24] showed that a 200-N posteriorly directed force did not cause posterior translation of the talus with up to 40% osteotomy

of posterolateral tibia, as long as the fibula and AITFL were intact. However, in tested cadavers, with transected AITFL and fibula, a significant posterior translation of the talus occurred after removal of 30% of the articular surface.

Harper and colleagues[25,26] showed that no significant posterior translation of the talus occurred even with a PMF measuring 50% of the articular surface. However, if the fibula is not intact or there is disruption of the lateral ligamentous structures, significant posterior translation of the talus occurred.

Macko and colleagues[20] showed with cadaver specimens that with increased size of the PMF to more than a third of the distal tibia, the surface area of contact decreased. Also, there were considerable changes in the load-distribution patterns, with increased confluence and concentration of loads as the size of the fragment increased. Similar findings were reported by Harttford and colleagues,[28] who showed a decrease in tibiotalar contact area with increasing size of posterior malleolus fragments. Also, sectioning of the deltoid ligament did not alter the contact area.

In contrast, Vrahas and colleagues[27] found that, even after removing 40% of the posterior malleolus, no increase in peak contact stress was detected. Similarly, Fitzpatrick and colleagues[29] studied dynamic contact stress aberrations in a cadaveric 50% PMF model. With dynamic range of motion, there was no increase in peak contact stress but a shift in the location of the contact stresses to a more anterior and medial location following the fracture. Furthermore, even in the anatomically fixated model, the stress redistribution did not return to normal. The investigators concluded that, with no talar subluxation and no increase in contact stresses near the articular incongruity, it is more likely that posttraumatic arthrosis is caused by the remaining articular surface being exposed to an increased stress. This shift in the center of stress loads cartilage that normally is exposed to little load.

In summary, conflicting data exist regarding the biomechanical influence of PMFs on ankle joint stability and contact pressures, especially in terms of fragment size.

RADIOGRAPHIC ASSESSMENT AND FRACTURE CLASSIFICATION

Conventional radiography is indicated for initial diagnosis and treatment of ankle fractures, with identification of posterior malleolar injury best evaluated on the lateral view.[30] Although the

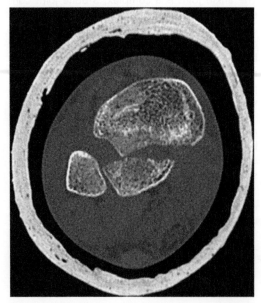

Fig. 1. Postmalleolus fracture with syndesmotic widening.

size of the posterior malleolar fragment can be estimated as a percentage of the tibial articular surface on the lateral view, several investigators have shown that radiograph-based measurement is poorly reliable and accurate.[31–34]

The authors recommend, in accordance with other studies, that computed tomography (CT) scan should be performed for all PMFs to evaluate fragment size, comminution, articular impaction, and syndesmotic disruption. Several investigators have shown that preoperative CT changed the surgeon's treatment and operative plan.[35,36]

Previous investigators classified PMFs based on the fragment size. However, this has been subjected to significant scrutiny. There is much debate on the correlation between fragment size and treatment indication. Haraguchi and colleagues[37] studied 57 cases of PMF. Based on preoperative CT scans, the investigators classified the fracture into 3 types: type I, the

posterolateral-oblique type (67% of cases); type II, the medial-extension type (19% of cases); and type III, the small-shell fragment (14% of cases) (Fig. 2). The investigators acknowledged that great variation in fracture patterns exists, and that preoperative use of CT scans may be justified. Mangnus and colleagues[38] performed CT-based PMF mapping in a series of 45 patients. They showed that there is a continuous spectrum of Haraguchi type III to I fractures and identified Haraguchi type II as a separate pattern. The investigators concluded that the morphology of the fracture might be more important than fragment size alone for clinical decision making.

Bartoníček and colleagues[39] suggested an alternative classification system. Based on CT scans, these investigators recognized 5 fracture patterns: type 1; extraincisural fragment with an intact fibular notch; type 2, posterolateral fragment extending into the fibular notch; type

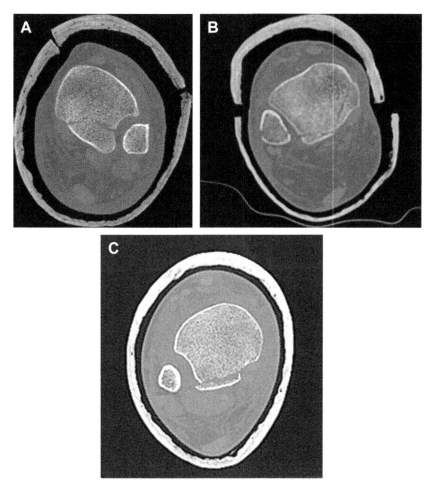

Fig. 2. Haraguchi classification of PMFs, based on CT axial images. (A) Type I, posterolateral oblique fragment. (B) Type II, medial-extension type. (C) Type III, small shell-shaped fragments at the posterior lip of the tibial plafond.

3, posteromedial 2-part fragment involving the medial malleolus; type 4, large posterolateral triangular fragment; and type 5, nonclassified, irregular, osteoporotic fragments.

Also, it is important to address the term posterior pilon variant. This fracture is characterized by an additional posteromedial fragment as well as comminution and marginal impaction.[40–42]

MANAGEMENT OF POSTERIOR MALLEOLAR FRACTURES

Principles of Treatment

Isolated, nondisplaced PMFs should be treated conservatively. Several investigators have shown that, with nonsurgical treatment of these fractures, satisfactory outcomes can be achieved.[30,43,44]

The indications for reduction and fixation of displaced PMFs remain controversial. In the past, the size of the posterior malleolar fragment was the main consideration for whether it should be addressed surgically. It was recommended that, if fragment size is greater than 25% to 33% of the articular surface, then it should be reduced and fixated.[20,23,28,45,46] However, this conception was based in part on biomechanical evidence of altered joint biomechanics and tibiotalar instability, rather than on the goal of restoring ankle joint stability and preventing posterior translation.

The authors suggest that surgical criteria for the reduction and fixation of the PMF should be based on the concept of restoring ankle joint structural integrity. The preoperative radiographs and CT scans should be thoroughly analyzed to formulate a good understanding of the specific fracture characteristics. Surgeons should assess the amount of articular incongruity caused by the posterior malleolar fragment, evidence of loose bodies and articular impaction, and whether the syndesmosis instability is caused by the fracture pattern (as shown, for example, in Fig. 1).

The posteromedial or posterolateral surgical approaches readily enable surgeons to address these components of the injury. Once lateral malleolus fracture is reduced, the posterior malleolar fragment is often reduced with ligamentotaxis of the PITFL. If this is not the case, and articular congruity is not achieved, this is an indication for reduction and fixation of the posterior fragment. Furthermore, if posterior talar translation persists, as judged by lateral fluoroscopy, then the posterior malleolar fragment should be addressed. In cases in which small osteochondral fragments may interfere with anatomic reduction or become loose bodies, or articular

impaction is recognized, then it is advisable to approach the fracture site and address this before attempting reduction and fixation of lateral malleolus fracture. In addition, assessing ankle joint syndesmotic and rotatory instability is of paramount importance, and is a major component of surgical indication. The effect of posterior malleolar fragment and PITFL on ankle joint syndesmotic and rotatory stability was emphasized and described earlier. The fixation of posterior malleolar fragments to achieve stability, thereby restoring ankle joint structural integrity, has been supported by several studies.[47,48] In a cadaveric study by Gardner and colleagues,[47] the investigators showed that, compared with intact specimens, syndesmotic stiffness was restored to 70% after fixation of the posterior malleolus and to 40% after syndesmotic screw fixation. This finding is supported by several investigators[48,49] comparing syndesmotic stabilization with trans-syndesmotic screw to posterior malleolar fixation/PITFL repair. The investigators concluded that direct posterior malleolar fixation or PITFL repair is at least equivalent to syndesmotic screw fixation.

Surgical Approach and Technique

Several surgical approaches are available for the treatment of PMFs. The type of the PMF, and the existence of medial and/or lateral malleolus fractures, are all considered in terms of approach and patient positioning.[50] Direct visualization of the posterior malleolar fragment can be achieved with posterior approaches to the ankle joint.

The posteromedial approach is appropriate for a posteromedial fragment, and allows concomitant treatment of the medial malleolus.[51–53] This approach is based on a skin incision that follows the posteromedial border of the distal tibia and medial malleolus and continues in line with the tibialis posterior tendon. Exposure of the tibia is made with deeper incision between the posterior tibialis tendon and flexor digitorum longus, or between both tendons and the neurovascular bundle. A retrospective study by Bois and colleagues[52] showed good short-term and midterm clinical results with the posteromedial approach and fracture buttress plate fixation of large posterior malleolar fragments (Fig. 3). The posterolateral approach has gained much popularity, and allows good visualization of the posterolateral malleolar fragment.[51,54–57] Furthermore, concomitant treatment of the fibula fracture is easily performed. Usually the patient is placed in a prone

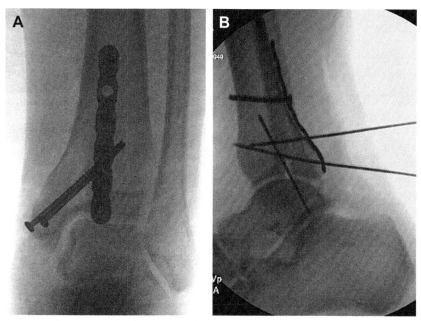

Fig. 3. (A,B) Fixation of posteromedial fragment performed via posteromedial approach.

position, and the skin incision is made midway between the lateral border of Achilles tendon and the posterior border of the fibula, or directly over the posteromedial border of the fibula. During superficial dissection, the sural nerve must be identified and protected where it courses through the surgical field.[58] The deep dissection develops the plane between the flexor hallucis longus (FHL) and peroneals. Once the FHL muscle belly is elevated from the fibula and lateral tibia, and retracted medially, the posterolateral fragment is visualized. While exposing and manipulating the fragment, great care should be taken to preserve the PITFL. Reduction is facilitated with dorsiflexion of the ankle. A ball spike or bone tamp aids in achieving reduction, and a temporary fixation with Kirschner wire can be performed, with reduction checked with fluoroscopy. Once the fragment is properly reduced, a slightly under-contoured plate can be used in an antiglide technique.[57] The fibula fracture can be addressed with mobilization of the peroneal tendons and posterior plating. Which fracture should be addressed first is a matter of debate. Although first fixating the fibula restores length and facilitates the posterior malleolar reduction, the fibular plate can hinder adequate visualization of the posterior malleolar reduction with fluoroscopy (Fig. 4). For these reasons, the authors' preferred technique is to address the fibula first. Once the length and fibular fracture

reduction is achieved, provisional fixation of the fibula is done with Kirschner wire or a reduction clamp. Attention is then given to the reduction and fixation of the posterior malleolus, without the interference of a fibular plate in fluoroscopy (Fig. 5). Only then is definitive fixation

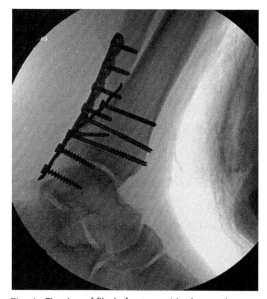

Fig. 4. Fixation of fibula fracture with plate and screws facilitates posterior malleolus fragment reduction, but makes it challenging to obtain adequate visualization of the fragment reduction.

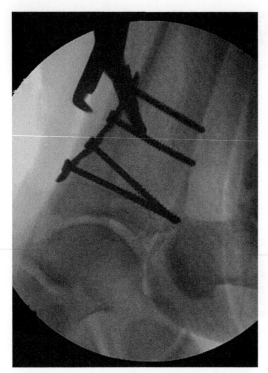

Fig. 5. Temporary reduction of fibula fracture with a reduction clamp aids posterior malleolar reduction and fixation, and enables confirmation of adequate posterior fragment reduction with fluoroscopy.

of the fibula performed. If fixation of the medial malleolus is required, it can be done with the patient in the prone position, or, if more complex medial malleolar fractures are present, the patient can be repositioned to the supine position. Alternatively, indirect reduction by ligamentotaxis of the PITFL can be attempted. However, this type of reduction cannot always ensure adequate articular reduction or treatment of impacted plafond or small osteochondral debris. The most common method of PMF fixation with this technique is with anterior-to-posterior (AP) screws. O'Connor and colleagues[59] compared patients who underwent posterior plating with patients who were treated with AP screw fixation and showed that patients treated with plating had superior clinical outcomes at follow-up compared with those treated with AP screws.

OUTCOMES AND PROGNOSIS

No consensus exists on the outcome and prognosis of PMFs. The current literature is fragmented in terms of methodology and outcome measures. Overall, trimalleolar fractures have worse prognosis compared with unimalleolar or bimalleolar fractures; that is, the presence of a posterior tibial component has an adverse effect on outcome.[60,61] Furthermore, there is evidence that, with posterior malleolar fragments greater than 25% to 33% of the articular surface, there is a higher risk for poor outcome.[45,62–65] However, as emphasized earlier, posterior malleolus fragment size should not be used as the sole criterion for the decision of surgical intervention. Langenhuijsen and colleagues[66] showed that achieving joint congruity with or without fixation was a significant factor in prognosis. They recommended reduction and fixation of fragments involving 10% or more of the articular surface that remained displaced adequate medial and lateral malleolus reduction. This recommendation is further supported by the work of Jaskulka and colleagues,[45] showing significantly better long-term results in posterior malleolar fragments involving greater than 5% of the articular surface treated surgically compared with those treated nonsurgically. A recent work by Evers and colleagues[67] showed that patients with fragments smaller than 25% of the distal tibial joint surface, which in most cases were not treated with osteosynthesis, had worse outcomes. In contrast, other investigators showed no difference in results with surgical and nonsurgical treatment of PMFs, even with fragments larger than 25% of the articular surface.[46,68–70] Xu and colleagues[69] showed no statistical differences in the American Orthopaedic Foot & Ankle Society and Visual Analog Scale scores among different fragment sizes. However, more advanced posttraumatic arthritis was correlated with larger fragment size. De Vries and colleagues[68] studied 45 patients with ankle fractures and posterior malleolar fragments. They showed that mean size of fixated posterior fragments was significantly larger than that of non-fixated fragments (30% vs 16%). Those patients in whom the PMF was fixated did not have a statistically significantly better outcome than those patients in whom the fragments were not fixated. The investigators concluded that there was no evidence for the need for fixation of fragments smaller than 25%. Drijfhout van Hooff and colleagues[70] conducted a retrospective study on 131 patients with PMFs. They found more radiographic osteoarthritis in patients with medium and large posterior fragments than in those with small fragments. Also, radiographic osteoarthritis occurred more frequently when postoperative step-off was 1 mm or more, whether the posterior fragment was fixed or not. However, clinical outcomes did not correlate with fragment size.

SUMMARY

PMFs are varied in morphology. A CT scan is imperative for the evaluation of fragment size, comminution, articular impaction, and syndesmotic disruption. Despite an increasing body of literature regarding PMFs, many questions remain unanswered. Although, historically, fragment size (25%–33% of articular surface) was considered a threshold for fixation, it is becoming evident that fragment size should not be the only factor to dictate treatment. Surgeons should focus on restoring ankle joint structural integrity; that is, restoring articular congruity, correcting posterior talar translation, addressing articular impaction, removing osteochondral debris, and achieving syndesmotic stability. Surgeons should familiarize themselves with posterolateral and posteromedial approaches and the technique of direct reduction and internal fixation in order to improve treatment outcomes.

REFERENCES

1. Court-Brown CM, McBirnie J, Wilson G. Adult ankle fractures–an increasing problem? Acta Orthop Scand 1998;69(1):43–7.
2. Kannus P, Palvanen M, Niemi S, et al. Increasing number and incidence of low-trauma ankle fractures in elderly people: Finnish statistics during 1970-2000 and projections for the future. Bone 2002;31(3):430–3.
3. Kannus P, Parkkari J, Niemi S, et al. Epidemiology of osteoporotic ankle fractures in elderly persons in Finland. Ann Intern Med 1996;125(12):975–8.
4. Kadakia RJ, Hsu RY, Hayda R, et al. Evaluation of one-year mortality after geriatric ankle fractures in patients admitted to nursing homes. Injury 2015; 46(10):2010–5.
5. Koval KJ, Lurie J, Zhou W, et al. Ankle fractures in the elderly: what you get depends on where you live and who you see. J Orthop Trauma 2005; 19(9):635–9.
6. Boraiah S, Gardner MJ, Helfet DL, et al. High association of posterior malleolus fractures with spiral distal tibial fractures. Clin Orthop Relat Res 2008; 466(7):1692–8.
7. Kukkonen J, Heikkilä JT, Kyyrönen T, et al. Posterior malleolar fracture is often associated with spiral tibial diaphyseal fracture: a retrospective study. J Trauma 2006;60(5):1058–60.
8. Fu S, Zou ZY, Mei G, et al. Advances and disputes of posterior malleolus fracture. Chin Med J (Engl) 2013;126(20):3972–7.
9. Irwin TA, Lien J, Kadakia AR. Posterior malleolus fracture. J Am Acad Orthop Surg 2013;21(1):32–40.
10. Odak S, Ahluwalia R, Unnikrishnan P, et al. Management of posterior malleolar fractures: a systematic review. J Foot Ankle Surg 2016;55(1):140–5.
11. van den Bekerom MP, Haverkamp D, Kloen P. Biomechanical and clinical evaluation of posterior malleolar fractures. A systematic review of the literature. J Trauma 2009;66(1):279–84.
12. Campbell KJ, Michalski MP, Wilson KJ, et al. The ligament anatomy of the deltoid complex of the ankle: a qualitative and quantitative anatomical study. J Bone Joint Surg Am 2014;96(8):e62.
13. Davidovitch RI, Egol KA. The medial malleolus osteoligamentous complex and its role in ankle fractures. Bull NYU Hosp Jt Dis 2009;67(4): 318–24.
14. Tochigi Y, Rudert MJ, Saltzman CL, et al. Contribution of articular surface geometry to ankle stabilization. J Bone Joint Surg Am 2006;88(12):2704–13.
15. van den Bekerom MP, Oostra RJ, Golanó P, et al. The anatomy in relation to injury of the lateral collateral ligaments of the ankle: a current concepts review. Clin Anat 2008;21(7):619–26.
16. Yablon IG, Heller FG, Shouse L. The key role of the lateral malleolus in displaced fractures of the ankle. J Bone Joint Surg Am 1977;59(2):169–73.
17. Henderson M. Trimalleolar fractures of the ankle. J Surg Clin North Am 1932;12:867–72.
18. Hermans JJ, Beumer A, de Jong TA, et al. Anatomy of the distal tibiofibular syndesmosis in adults: a pictorial essay with a multimodality approach. J Anat 2010;217(6):633–45.
19. Ogilvie-Harris DJ, Reed SC, Hedman TP. Disruption of the ankle syndesmosis: biomechanical study of the ligamentous restraints. Arthroscopy 1994; 10(5):558–60.
20. Macko VW, Matthews LS, Zwirkoski P, et al. The joint-contact area of the ankle. The contribution of the posterior malleolus. J Bone Joint Surg Am 1991;73(3):347–51.
21. Calhoun JH, Ledbetter BR, Viegas SF, et al. A comprehensive study of pressure distribution in the ankle joint with inversion and eversion. Foot Ankle Int 1994;15(3):125–33.
22. Lundberg A, Svensson OK, Németh G, et al. The axis of rotation of the ankle joint. J Bone Joint Surg Br 1989;71(1):94–9.
23. Scheidt KB, Stiehl JB, Skrade DA, et al. Posterior malleolar ankle fractures: an in vitro biomechanical analysis of stability in the loaded and unloaded states. J Orthop Trauma 1992;6(1):96–101.
24. Raasch WG, Larkin JJ, Draganich LF. Assessment of the posterior malleolus as a restraint to posterior subluxation of the ankle. J Bone Joint Surg Am 1992;74(8):1201–6.
25. Harper MC. Talar shift. The stabilizing role of the medial, lateral, and posterior ankle structures. Clin Orthop Relat Res 1990;(257):177–83.

26. Harper MC. Posterior instability of the talus: an anatomic evaluation. Foot Ankle 1989;10(1):36–9.

27. Vrahas M, Fu F, Veenis B. Intraarticular contact stresses with simulated ankle malunions. J Orthop Trauma 1994;8(2):159–66.

28. Hartford JM, Gorczyca JT, McNamara JL, et al. Tibiotalar contact area. Contribution of posterior malleolus and deltoid ligament. Clin Orthop Relat Res 1995;(320):182–7.

29. Fitzpatrick DC, Otto JK, McKinley TO, et al. Kinematic and contact stress analysis of posterior malleolus fractures of the ankle. J Orthop Trauma 2004;18(5):271–8.

30. Neumaier Probst E, Maas R, Meenen NM. Isolated fracture of the posterolateral tibial lip (Volkmann's triangle). Acta Radiol 1997;38(3):359–62.

31. Ferries JS, DeCoster TA, Firoozbakhsh KK, et al. Plain radiographic interpretation in trimalleolar ankle fractures poorly assesses posterior fragment size. J Orthop Trauma 1994;8(4):328–31.

32. Ebraheim NA, Mekhail AO, Haman SP. External rotation-lateral view of the ankle in the assessment of the posterior malleolus. Foot Ankle Int 1999; 20(6):379–83.

33. Buchler L, Tannast M, Bonel HM, et al. Reliability of radiologic assessment of the fracture anatomy at the posterior tibial plafond in malleolar fractures. J Orthop Trauma 2009;23(3):208–12.

34. Meijer DT, Doornberg JN, Sierevelt IN, et al. Guesstimation of posterior malleolar fractures on lateral plain radiographs. Injury 2015;46(10):2024–9.

35. Meijer DT, de Muinck Keizer RJ, Doornberg JN, et al. Diagnostic accuracy of 2-dimensional computed tomography for articular involvement and fracture pattern of posterior malleolar fractures. Foot Ankle Int 2016;37(1):75–82.

36. Palmanovich E, Brin YS, Laver L, et al. The effect of minimally displaced posterior malleolar fractures on decision making in minimally displaced lateral malleolus fractures. Int Orthop 2014;38(5):1051–6.

37. Haraguchi N, Haruyama H, Toga H, et al. Pathoanatomy of posterior malleolar fractures of the ankle. J Bone Joint Surg Am 2006;88(5):1085–92.

38. Mangnus L, Meijer DT, Stufkens SA, et al. Posterior malleolar fracture patterns. J Orthop Trauma 2015; 29(9):428–35.

39. Bartonicek J, Rammelt S, Kostlivý K, et al. Anatomy and classification of the posterior tibial fragment in ankle fractures. Arch Orthop Trauma Surg 2015; 135(4):505–16.

40. Karachalios T, Roidis N, Karoutis D, et al. Trimalleolar fracture with a double fragment of the posterior malleolus: a case report and modified operative approach to internal fixation. Foot Ankle Int 2001; 22(2):144–9.

41. Weber M. Trimalleolar fractures with impaction of the posteromedial tibial plafond: implications

for talar stability. Foot Ankle Int 2004;25(10): 716–27.

42. Gardner MJ, Streubel PN, McCormick JJ, et al. Surgeon practices regarding operative treatment of posterior malleolus fractures. Foot Ankle Int 2011; 32(4):385–93.

43. Donken CC, Goorden AJ, Verhofstad MH, et al. The outcome at 20 years of conservatively treated 'isolated' posterior malleolar fractures of the ankle: a case series. J Bone Joint Surg Br 2011;93(12): 1621–5.

44. Nugent JF, Gale BD. Isolated posterior malleolar ankle fractures. J Foot Surg 1990;29(1):80–3.

45. Jaskulka RA, Ittner G, Schedl R. Fractures of the posterior tibial margin: their role in the prognosis of malleolar fractures. J Trauma 1989;29(11):1565–70.

46. Harper MC, Hardin G. Posterior malleolar fractures of the ankle associated with external rotation-abduction injuries. Results with and without internal fixation. J Bone Joint Surg Am 1988;70(9):1348–56.

47. Gardner MJ, Brodsky A, Briggs SM, et al. Fixation of posterior malleolar fractures provides greater syndesmotic stability. Clin Orthop Relat Res 2006; 447:165–71.

48. Miller AN, Carroll EA, Parker RJ, et al. Posterior malleolar stabilization of syndesmotic injuries is equivalent to screw fixation. Clin Orthop Relat Res 2010;468(4):1129–35.

49. Schottel PC, Baxter J, Gilbert S, et al. Anatomic ligament repair restores ankle and syndesmotic rotational stability as much as syndesmotic screw fixation. J Orthop Trauma 2016;30(2):e36–40.

50. Wang X, Ma X, Zhang C, et al. Anatomical factors affecting the selection of an operative approach for fibular fractures involving the posterior malleolus. Exp Ther Med 2013;5(3):757–60.

51. Amorosa LF, Brown GD, Greisberg J. A surgical approach to posterior pilon fractures. J Orthop Trauma 2010;24(3):188–93.

52. Bois AJ, Dust W. Posterior fracture dislocation of the ankle: technique and clinical experience using a posteromedial surgical approach. J Orthop Trauma 2008;22(9):629–36.

53. Mizel MS, Temple HT. Technique tip: revisit to a surgical approach to allow direct fixation of fractures of the posterior and medial malleolus. Foot Ankle Int 2004;25(6):440–2.

54. Abdelgawad AA, Kadous A, Kanlic E. Posterolateral approach for treatment of posterior malleolus fracture of the ankle. J Foot Ankle Surg 2011;50(5): 607–11.

55. Forberger J, Sabandal PV, Dietrich M, et al. Posterolateral approach to the displaced posterior malleolus: functional outcome and local morbidity. Foot Ankle Int 2009;30(4):309–14.

56. Franzone JM, Vosseller JT. Posterolateral approach for open reduction and internal fixation of a

posterior malleolus fracture–hinging on an intact PITFL to disimpact the tibial plafond: a technical note. Foot Ankle Int 2013;34(8):1177–81.

57. Tornetta P 3rd, Ricci W, Nork S, et al. The postero-lateral approach to the tibia for displaced posterior malleolar injuries. J Orthop Trauma 2011;25(2): 123–6.

58. Jowett AJ, Sheikh FT, Carare RO, et al. Location of the sural nerve during posterolateral approach to the ankle. Foot Ankle Int 2010;31(10):880–3.

59. O'Connor TJ, Mueller B, Ly TV, et al. "A to P" screw versus posterolateral plate for posterior malleolus fixation in trimalleolar ankle fractures. J Orthop Trauma 2015;29(4):e151–6.

60. Verhage SM, Schipper IB, Hoogendoorn JM. Long-term functional and radiographic outcomes in 243 operated ankle fractures. J Foot Ankle Res 2015;8:45.

61. Tejwani NC, Pahk B, Egol KA. Effect of posterior malleolus fracture on outcome after unstable ankle fracture. J Trauma 2010;69(3):666–9.

62. Mingo-Robinet J, López-Durán L, Galeote JE, et al. Ankle fractures with posterior malleolar fragment: management and results. J Foot Ankle Surg 2011; 50(2):141–5.

63. McDaniel WJ, Wilson FC. Trimalleolar fractures of the ankle. An end result study. Clin Orthop Relat Res 1977;(122):37–45.

64. Lindsjo U. Operative treatment of ankle fracture-dislocations. A follow-up study of 306/321 consec-utive cases. Clin Orthop Relat Res 1985;(199): 28–38.

65. Broos PL, Bisschop AP. Operative treatment of ankle fractures in adults: correlation between types of fracture and final results. Injury 1991; 22(5):403–6.

66. Langenhuijsen JF, Heetveld MJ, Ultee JM, et al. Re-sults of ankle fractures with involvement of the pos-terior tibial margin. J Trauma 2002;53(1):55–60.

67. Evers J, Barz L, Wähnert D, et al. Size matters: the influence of the posterior fragment on patient out-comes in trimalleolar ankle fractures. Injury 2015; 46(Suppl 4):S109–13.

68. De Vries JS, Wijgman AJ, Sierevelt IN, et al. Long-term results of ankle fractures with a posterior mal-leolar fragment. J Foot Ankle Surg 2005;44(3): 211–7.

69. Xu HL, Li X, Zhang DY, et al. A retrospective study of posterior malleolus fractures. Int Orthop 2012; 36(9):1929–36.

70. Drijfhout van Hooff CC, Verhage SM, Hoogendoorn JM. Influence of fragment size and postoperative joint congruency on long-term outcome of posterior malleolar fractures. Foot Ankle Int 2015;36(6):673–8.

Current Controversies in Management of Calcaneus Fractures

Heather E. Gotha, MD, Jacob R. Zide, MD*

KEYWORDS

- Calcaneus fracture • Subtalar arthritis • Sinus tarsi approach • Peroneal displacement

---

KEY POINTS

- Contrary to previous teaching, the "constant fragment" may be displaced, especially in more comminuted fractures with medial extension across the posterior facet.
- Restoration of Bohler's angle (BA) intraoperatively, regardless of the angle at presentation, may be a better predictor of patient outcomes over time.
- Sanders type III and IV fractures requiring later subtalar arthrodesis had better outcomes and fewer wound complications after arthrodesis if they had originally undergone open reduction and internal fixation (ORIF).
- The sinus tarsi approach for ORIF of calcaneus fractures is gaining in popularity and is associated with fewer wound complications in most settings.
- Operative management with near-anatomic reduction of the posterior facet and restoration of overall calcaneal morphology offers greater potential for superior short- and long-term outcomes.

INTRODUCTION

The optimal treatment of displaced intraarticular calcaneus fractures (DIACFs) remains a subject of debate among orthopedic surgeons. These fractures account for nearly 75% of all calcaneus fractures[1] and are associated with unpredictable, and relatively poor, short- and long-term clinical outcomes. The social and economic impact of DIACFS is substantial on both an individual and societal level. The overwhelming majority of these fractures tend to involve young males, many of whom—an estimated 55%—earn a living by performing manual labor. Many remain incapacitated for 3 to 5 years after injury, and never return to their preinjury employment or level of activity. Analysis of Short Form (SF)-36 scores of these patients at 2 years after injury has demonstrated similar functional levels to those of patients who underwent organ transplantation or suffered from myocardial infarction.[2,3]

Prospective, randomized trials concerning the management of DIACFs have shown somewhat equivocal results of operative versus nonoperative treatment.[3–5] However, more recent trends in the literature (particularly recent metaanalyses and longer term follow-up studies) have suggested that anatomic reduction and stable fixation results in better outcomes in terms of early restoration of function, patient satisfaction, minimization of symptomatic posttraumatic arthritis, and better results of subtalar fusion in the setting of posttraumatic arthritis.[6–9]

Unfortunately, there is no "one-size-fits-all" approach to the operative management of calcaneus fractures, nor is there a "one size fits many" approach. DIACFs pose unique and complex challenges from an operative standpoint, even for the experienced orthopedic surgeon. Careful

---

The authors have nothing to disclose.
Department of Orthopaedic Surgery, Baylor University Medical Center, 3900 Junius Street, Suite 500, Dallas, TX 75246, USA
* Corresponding author.
E-mail address: Jacob.Zide@BSWHealth.org

consideration of soft tissue characteristics, fracture pattern, timing of surgery, surgical approach, and patient demographics is essential to optimizing outcomes in theses fractures. Additionally, the surgeon must be aware of and prepared to treat concurrent pathology that has a tendency to be overlooked at the time of initial injury—specifically calcaneocuboid joint (CCJ) involvement and peroneal tendon dislocation.

ANATOMIC CONSIDERATIONS

An understanding of the anatomy of the calcaneus and its surrounding structures is critical to understanding mechanisms of fracture, characteristic fracture patterns, surgical approaches, and long-term sequela of injury.

The calcaneus is the largest and the most frequently fractured tarsal bone. It has several soft tissue attachments that render it integral to weight-bearing and overall gait mechanics. The Achilles tendon attaches to the posterior inferior aspect of the calcaneal tuberosity, which allows the calcaneus to serve as the primary lever arm for the triceps surae and facilitate the transmission of force from the hindfoot to the midfoot and forefoot during gait. At the same time, the calcaneus maintains the length of the lateral column and protects the posteromedial arch contents.

The calcaneus has 4 key articulations with surrounding structures. Superiorly, the calcaneus shares 3 articulating surfaces with the talus—the anterior, middle, and posterior facets of the subtalar joint. The posterior facet is largest of the 3 articulations and forms the primary load-bearing component of the subtalar joint. Its surface is convex and runs distally and laterally at approximately 45° to the sagittal plane. The fourth articulation lies at the distal end of the anterior process of the calcaneus and forms the CCJ.

The sustentaculum tali protrudes from the medial aspect of the calcaneal body and provides a shelf of dense cortical bone to support the talar neck. The superomedial spring ligament—a key supporter of the arch and talar neck—originates here, along with the tibiocalcaneal component of the deltoid ligament—a key ankle stabilizer.

These robust soft tissue attachments, along with the interosseous talocalcaneal ligaments, are what have historically led to the sustentaculum being described as the "constant fragment," because these attachments were thought to keep the sustentaculum tightly bound to the talus, and thus in a relatively constant position. Traditionally, open reduction and internal fixation (ORIF) through extensile lateral approach has involved reducing the remaining fragments of the calcaneus back to the nondisplaced sustentacular fragment.

However, recent literature has called into question the "constancy" of this fragment in DIACFs, particularly in more comminuted fractures with more medial extension across the posterior facet. In a 2013 study, Berberian and colleagues[10] retrospectively reviewed the computed tomography (CT) scans of 88 patients with 100 DIACFs for evidence of sustentacular displacement and/or angulation. Gapping and intraarticular displacement of the middle facet was also examined and included in the definition of sustentacular displacement. The authors found that the sustentaculum was displaced in 42 of these fractures. Fractures involving more than 50% of the posterior facet (consistent with Sanders B and C type fractures) as well as 3 and 4 part fractures of the posterior facet were found to have significant association with sustentacular displacement. Similarly, Gitajn and colleagues[11] found sustentacular fractures in 94 of 212 calcaneal fractures. Of these 94 sustentacular fractures, 20.3% (n = 43) demonstrated subluxation of the articulation between the sustentaculum and the talus.

Overall, as these recent studies suggest, the surgeon must pay special attention to the alignment and integrity of the "constant" fragment—particularly in those DIACFs that involve the medial aspect of the posterior facet. In cases in which the constant fragment is angulated or subluxated, it has been suggested combined medial and lateral approaches be used, although the data to support this remain scant[12–14] (Fig. 1). Importantly, however, no studies to date have directly assessed the utility of a combined medial and lateral approach in the reduction of a displaced sustentacular fracture in the setting of a DIACF.

MECHANISM OF INJURY AND PATHOANATOMY

Intraarticular calcaneal fractures occur after eccentric axial loading of the talus on the calcaneus, typically as a result of high-energy mechanism such as motor vehicle collision or fall from height. This axial loading drives the lateral border of the talus into the body of the calcaneus, creating a shear fracture through the posterior facet, resulting in medial and lateral fragments. The position of the subtalar joint during axial loading determines how medial or lateral this split occurs. As originally described by Essex-Lopresti, the classic primary fracture

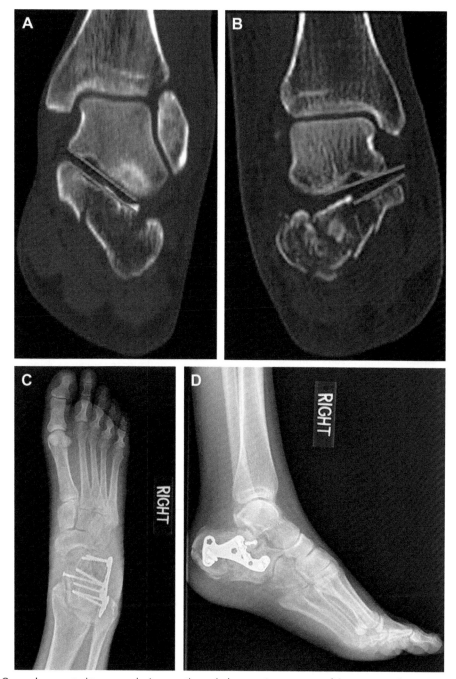

Fig. 1. Coronal computed tomography images through the anterior-most cut of the posterior facet, demonstrating a nondisplaced sustentacular fragment (A), and an angulated fragment (B). (C, D) Fixation of the fragment in B with a single lag screw directed from medial to lateral.

line runs from anterolateral to posteromedial. As the axial load continues to be applied, secondary fracture lines extend from the primary shear line. A posteriorly directed load drives the fracture line into and posterior to the posterior facet, thus separating the posterior facet and the tuberosity. The tuberosity tilts into varus and equinus as a result of the pull of the triceps surae. The posterior facet fragment is then driven into the calcaneal body, resulting in a joint depression–type fracture. As the body of the talus drives the posterior facet fragment further into the cancellous calcaneal body, it shears the attachment of the posterior facet fragment from the lateral wall, and results in lateral wall blowout.[15,16]

Overall, this mechanism tends to result in a characteristic pattern of displacement in joint depression–type DIACFs. If managed nonoperatively or malreduced, a typical constellation of findings and disabling long-term sequelae often result (Fig. 2).

- The disruption of the posterior facet and residual surface incongruity, over time, results in painful posttraumatic subtalar arthritis.
- The expansion of the lateral wall owing to lateral wall blowout leads to heel widening, which can cause difficulty with shoe wear, subfibular impingement, peroneal stenosis, tendonitis, and possible dislocation.
- Loss of the talar declination angle, which occurs as a result of loss of calcaneal body height (as represented by a decreased BA), results in anterior tibiotalar impingement, and decreased ankle dorsiflexion.
- Residual varus of the calcaneal tuberosity leads to overall hindfoot varus, causing painful lateral column overload.

IMAGING AND CLASSIFICATION OF INJURY

Initial radiographic evaluation of calcaneal fractures should include anteroposterior, oblique, and lateral images of the foot. Standard imaging of the ankle should be included as well. Specialty views—such as Harris axial view of the heel and Broden's views of the posterior facet—may be obtained; however, many investigators have suggested that these views may be omitted as part of initial workup and preoperative planning if a CT scan is obtained.[17]

BA and the crucial angle of Gissane are useful radiographic parameters to define the severity of initial injury. BA is measured by a line connecting the highest point of the anterior process to the highest point of the posterior facet, and a line tangential to the superior edge of the tuberosity. Normal values for BA range from 20° to 40°, and a decrease in this angle suggests collapse of the posterior facet and overall loss of calcaneal height. The crucial angle of Gissane is formed by the dense subchondral bone of the posterior and anterior and middle facets; normal values are 120° to 145°.

The BA at the time of presentation has been acknowledged widely to correlate with injury severity; however, its prognostic value in terms of predicting morbidity associated with calcaneal fractures continues to remain a subject of debate. Significant loss of calcaneal height—as measured by initial BA of less than 0° on injury radiographs—has been shown in some studies to be predictive of poor outcomes and the need for late subtalar fusion, regardless of the type of treatment.[3,18] This correlation recently has been called into question, and newer literature has suggested that restoration of BA intraoperatively, regardless of the initial angle, may be a better predictor of patient outcomes over time. In a review of 274 patients with calcaneal fractures, Su and colleagues[19] found no correlation between

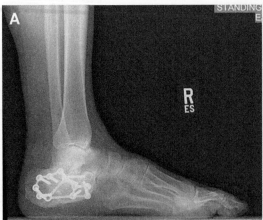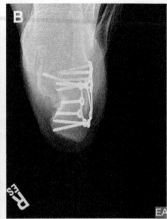

Fig. 2. Lateral and axial radiographs depicting classic sequelae of calcaneal fracture malreduction including severe posttraumatic arthritis of the subtalar with loss of talar declination angle and anterior tibiotalar impingement (A) as well as persistent lateral wall expansion and heel varus (B).

preoperative BA and postoperative function. Similarly, in a post hoc analysis of 2013 randomized, controlled trial comparing operative versus nonoperative treatment for DIACFs, Agren and colleagues[7] found no association between the pretreatment BA and outcomes. Both studies, however, found a correlation between BA at the time of healing and superior functional recovery.

CT has vastly enhanced the current understanding of the pathoanatomy of calcaneal fractures, and has become an integral component in management. The coronal views allow visualization of the articular fragments of the posterior facet, the sustentaculum, the extent of widening of the calcaneal body and lateral wall blow out, angulation of the tuberosity, and position of the FHL and peroneal tendons. On sagittal imaging, the rotational and inferior displacement of the posterior facet fragments can be visualized, along with the extent of involvement of the anterior process region and superior displacement of the tuberosity relative to the posterior facet (eg, overall loss of calcaneal height.) Axial views can reveal extension of the fracture into the anterior process and calcaneocuboi joint, as well as sustentaculum and anteroinferior posterior facet. Analysis of axial cuts at the level of the distal fibula can reveal dislocation or subluxation of the peroneal tendons.

The Sanders classification, which is the most commonly used system for the classification of calcaneus fractures, is based on the number and location of the articular fragments of the posterior facet. This system uses a coronal CT image through the widest portion of the posterior facet; roman numerals I though IV are used to indicate the number of fragments; the fragments are then subclassified further by letter designation (A, B, C) to denote the location of the primary fracture line from lateral to medial. Type A represent a lateral fracture line, type B is through the middle of the facet, and type C denotes a medial fracture line through the sustentaculum.[20]

The prognostic value of the Sanders classification of DIACFs has been heavily evaluated both in terms of short- and long-term outcomes, and the findings of these studies have become a critical component of surgical decision making and management recommendations.[3,21] Sanders type III and IV fractures, which involve more significant articular comminution, are more often associated with higher energy of injury. These fractures, therefore, involve not only greater disruption of soft tissues, but also overall disruption of calcaneal shape and morphology (and are more likely to have concurrent pathology, such as calcaneocuboid disruption and peroneal dislocation). It follows that Sanders type III and IV fractures have poorer results with nonoperative management compared with lower energy Sanders type II fractures.[3] Additionally, reflecting the significant articular damage associated with these injuries, it has been shown that operatively treated Sanders type III and IV fractures have a poorer prognosis, in terms of both function and need for late subtalar fusion, than operatively treated Sanders type II fractures.[22] Overall, regardless of treatment, patients with Sanders type IV fractures are nearly 6 times more likely to eventually require arthrodesis than patients with a Sanders type II fracture.[18]

CONTROVERSIES IN MANAGEMENT
Operative Versus Nonoperative Treatment
To date, the literature concerning the management of these fractures has been somewhat equivocal in terms of the benefits of operative treatment over nonoperative treatment. Historically, the unpredictable outcomes associated with ORIF, as well as high rate of complications, led many to advocate nonoperative care of these fractures.[23–25] As techniques of fracture care evolved, operative intervention for DIACFs became the treatment of choice at many orthopedic trauma centers.[20,26]

However, the landmark 2002 study published by Buckley and colleagues,[3] which is the largest randomized controlled clinical trial to date, seemed to again suggest limited benefit to ORIF from a functional standpoint. This large multicenter, randomized, controlled trial compared outcomes of operative versus nonoperative treatment of 471 DIACFs. The authors found no difference in total SF-36 and visual analog scale (VAS) scores between those patients treated operatively versus nonoperatively at a minimum follow-up of 2 years.

Some benefit to operative intervention was suggested, however. The authors reported a significant difference in the rate of arthrodesis between the operative and nonoperative group (7 of 206 vs 37 of 218; P = .001). Subgroup analysis excluding those patients receiving Workers' Compensation suggested that patients with a BA of 0° to 14°, a light workload, Sanders type II fracture, female gender, and age less than 30 years all benefitted from operative intervention and had higher SF-36 scores than their nonoperatively treated counterparts.[3] Csizy and colleagues[18] echoed these findings, noting that patients treated nonoperatively were 6 times more likely to require subtalar fusion than those treated with initial ORIF.

A subsequent economic evaluation of this same cohort by Brauer and colleagues[8] suggested operative treatment of DIACFs was economically advantageous compared with nonoperative management. This study estimated the direct health care costs and indirect costs associated with operative versus nonoperative treatment at a 4-year time horizon. Pertinent findings included a lower rate of subtalar arthrodesis associated with operative treatment, as well as shorter duration of time off work. When indirect costs (specifically estimated costs of time lost from work) were included, operative treatment was found to be significantly less costly and more effective in terms of minimizing need for future intervention.

Although there is little debate regarding the superior outcomes of operative treatment for simple DIACFs with articular stepoff but minimal comminution (eg, Sanders type II), the lack of a statistically significant improvement in functional outcomes with ORIF of Sanders type III and IV fractures, as well as associated risk of wound complication and infection, has led some to advocate nonoperative management of these more highly comminuted injuries.[4,5,18] Much of the recent literature, however, seems to suggest that restoration of overall calcaneal shape, alignment and height, which avoids many sequelae of calcaneal fracture malunion, confers a long-term functional benefit and may result in decreased rates of symptomatic subtalar arthritis.[7,19] Moreover, it has been shown that, in those patients with Sanders type III and IV who do go on to require subtalar arthrodesis, those who were treated with initial ORIF had better outcomes and fewer wound complications after arthrodesis than those patients initially managed nonoperatively. This reflects the extreme technical difficulty in restoring calcaneal height and the talocalcaneal relationship in patients with calcaneal malunion as result of initial nonoperative treatment.[9,27]

Acceptable nonoperative treatment criteria with regard to fracture pattern include those fractures that are truly nondisplaced, or those that have less than 2 mm of articular surface displacement. Additionally, the overall height, length, and width the calcaneus should be well-preserved. Finally, there should not be gross varus or valgus alignment of the tuberosity.[21]

Primary Open Reduction and Internal Fixation Plus Fusion Versus Open Reduction and Internal Fixation for Sanders Type IV Fractures

The optimal initial operative management of Sanders type IV fractures remains a subject of debate. The need for subsequent subtalar fusion for treatment of posttraumatic arthritis in operatively treated Sanders IV injuries has been reported to be as high as 73%, compared with 23% for Sanders III fractures.[28,29] Secondary surgeries to address painful posttraumatic arthritis increase both direct and indirect costs of care, and delay return to prior levels of function for the patient. In light of this, it has been argued that avoidance of a second surgery by initial treatment with primary ORIF and subtalar fusion is a more ideal treatment for patients with Sanders type IV fractures.[22] This has not yet been substantiated in the literature. A recent multicenter randomized trial comparing primary ORIF alone with primary ORIF with subtalar fusion showed no difference between the 2 treatment modalities in terms of functional outcomes.[30]

It is the experience of these authors that simultaneous restoration of calcaneal alignment and arthrodesis is a technically challenging operation. Attempting to obtain adequate compression across a comminuted posterior facet surface has the potential to result in calcaneal shortening, loss of height, and loss of alignment—regardless of the position before fusion. Furthermore, because much of the literature has demonstrated that not all posttraumatic subtalar arthritis is sufficiently symptomatic so as to require fusion, we suggest that ORIF be the initial treatment (when operative intervention is not contraindicated owing to other factors), and that patients be monitored postoperatively for the development of symptomatic subtalar arthritis. Restoring appropriate calcaneal height, length, and alignment at the time of the index surgery will allow for relatively simple and reliable in situ fusion at a later date.

Operative Approaches, Techniques, and Controversies

Extensile versus "minimally invasive"

A multitude of surgical approaches have been described in operative treatment of DACFs. Careful consideration of patient factors, fracture pattern, and timing of surgery—along with surgeon experience—are all essential to achieving optimal patient outcome while minimizing risk of complications.

The traditional approach for ORIF of DIACFs involves an extensile L-shaped lateral approach to the calcaneus. This approach has been the most frequently used surgical approach for the last 3 decades with which to reliably achieve anatomic reduction and restore width, height, and alignment, with placement of appropriate plate and screw fixation. The extensile lateral approach has also been noted to provide excellent fracture exposure, both of the posterior facet and lateral wall, and thus is preferable for more complex fractures.[21,31,32]

Although this approach offers excellent fracture visualization, it has been associated with rates of wound complication and infection as high as 20% to 37%.[33] Devascularization of the fracture fragments, larger surgical field, increased operative time, creation of potential dead space, and disruption of the lateral calcaneal branch of the peroneal artery (the primary vascular supply to the overlying fasciocutaneous flap) have all been hypothesized to contribute to this increase rate of complications.[34]

Recently, the sinus tarsi approach has been advocated as an alternative to the traditional lateral extensile approach. As most commonly described, this approach involves a 2- to 4-cm incision over the sinus tarsi, along a line from the tip of the fibula to the base of the fourth metatarsal. When performed appropriately, this approach allows for excellent visualization of the posterior facet, anterolateral fragment, CCJ, lateral wall, and peroneal tendons. If need be, the incision can be extended proximally to treat acute peroneal tendon dislocation. Likewise, the same incision can be used at a later date should subtalar arthrodesis or tendon debridement be indicated.

Proponents of the sinus tarsi approach cite such advantages as decreased operative time, minimization of soft tissue disruption, and fewer wound complications. In a retrospective review of 112 operatively treated calcaneus fractures (79 treated with lateral extensile approach and 33 with sinus tarsi), Kline and colleagues[35] found a significantly lower rate of wound complications in the sinus tarsi group (6%) compared with the lateral extensile group (29%; P = .005). Patients undergoing ORIF via an extensile lateral approach were also more likely to require secondary surgery within the 3-year study period, with 20% of patients requiring return to the operating room for varying indications. Importantly, fracture severity was relatively equally distributed among the 2 groups, with 53% Sanders type II fractures and 47% Sanders type III fractures in the extensile cohort, and 61% Sanders type II fractures and 39% Sanders type III fractures in the sinus tarsi cohort. Similarly, there were no differences between the 2 groups in terms of sex, age, tobacco use, or diabetes. Both groups had 100% union rate, with no measured differences in the final postoperative Bohlers angle and angle of Gissane.

A 2014 randomized prospective trial by Xia and colleagues[36] showed similar findings. In this study, 117 calcaneal fractures were allocated randomly to ORIF via lateral extensile approach versus sinus tarsi approach. All surgeries were performed 8 to 12 days after injury and used a titanium alloy low profile plate. The authors reported significantly decreased operative times in the sinus tarsi group compared with the extensile group (62 vs 93 minutes), as well as lower rate of wound complication (0% vs 16.3%). Although postoperative radiographic parameters of calcaneal reduction were equivalent for the 2 groups, patients in the minimally invasive group had significantly higher Maryland foot scores at the time of final follow-up.

Although much of the recent literature supports the utilization off the sinus tarsi approach in Sanders types II and III fractures,[37,38] few studies have investigated the use and complications of this approach in highly comminuted Sanders type IV fractures. Kwon and colleagues[39] recently conducted a retrospective review of 405 operatively treated DIACFs in which they examined risk of wound complications with regard to such factors as fracture severity, operative approach, and time to fixation. Although the authors found a decreased overall risk of wound complications with minimally invasive approaches (percutaneous and sinus tarsi techniques) compared with the extensile approach, they did note an increased risk of wound complication in Sanders types III and IV fractures treated with minimally invasive approaches compared with Sanders types I and fractures II treated with similar approach (odds ratio, 3.5; 95% confidence interval, 1.3–10.3; P = .018). Other pertinent findings included an increased risk of wound complication with operative delay beyond 14 days when using minimally invasive approaches (odds ratio, 3.2; 95% confidence interval, 1.3–9.5; P = .01).

However, these results should be interpreted with some caution. The outcomes of 24 different surgeons with varying degrees of operative experience were reviewed in this study, and the operative volumes of each individual surgeon are not reported. Additionally, the authors make no distinction between "minimally invasive" percutaneous techniques and "sinus tarsi" approach in their outcomes analysis. In the absence of standardized operative technique and surgeon experience, conclusions regarding specific complications of the sinus tarsi approach are limited.

Several other minimally invasive methods of operative fixation have been described, including percutaneous as well as arthroscopically assisted techniques. A limited number of retrospective studies and case series regarding percutaneous fixation techniques have been published, all of which demonstrate mixed results in terms of wound complication, quality of articular reduction, and patient outcomes.[40,41] Similarly, there is limited literature supporting routine use of arthroscopic-assisted reduction of the posterior facet in conjunction with percutaneous fixation techniques.[42–45]

Restoration of articular surfaces: importance of the posterior facet and calcaneocuboid joint

The importance of restoring the anatomy of the posterior facet in DIACFs, when possible, is well-documented. In their 2002 randomized, controlled trial, Buckley[3] and associates noted that, in patients not receiving workers' compensation, both anatomic reduction of the posterior facet and reduction with articular stepoff of less than 2 mm were associated with better overall SF-36 scores as well as VAS scores compared with those fractures with articular comminution.[3] However, the "comminuted" group in this analysis also included all non–workers' compensation patients treated nonoperatively. Thus, the results are somewhat misleading and ignore confounding variables that are addressed by operative fixation. These variables include restoration of calcaneal height, realignment of tuberosity, and reduction of lateral wall.

Later studies, however, have better supported the association between posterior facet reduction and improved functional outcomes. In a post hoc analysis of a 2013 randomized, controlled trial comparing operative versus nonoperative treatment for DIACFs, Agren and colleagues[7] noted that residual displacement of the articular surface was associated with lower AOFAS hindfoot score, VAS pain score, and Olerud-Molander score.

More recently, reduction of the calcaneocuboid surface has been suggested to be important to optimization of outcomes and restoration of lateral column function. The incidence of CCJ involvement in calcaneus fractures has been reported to be around 50%, ranging from 33% to 76%, depending on the series.[46–49] Multiple analyses have shown CCJ involvement to be more common in fractures of higher severity, particularly joint depression–type fractures involving lateral wall comminution and lateral subluxation of the posterior facet (Fig. 3). Despite this, a correlation between CCJ involvement and clinical outcomes has not yet been definitively established in the literature. In a comparative analysis outcomes of DIACFs involving the CCJ versus those that did not, Gallino and colleagues[47] found no difference in VAS and SF-36 scores at a mean of 2.3 years postoperatively. Additionally, although the severity of initial CCJ injury was found to correlate with increased incidence of posttraumatic arthritic changes, there was no difference in outcome scores between those patients with CCJ arthritis and those without. This finding echoed the findings of previous work by Hutchinson and Huebner.[49]

However, a later study by Kinner and colleagues[48] suggested that involvement of the CCJ played a more significant role in functional outcomes. In this study involving a cohort of 44 DIACFs, the authors found that patients with a postoperative stepoff or gap of the CCJ greater than 2 mm had significantly worse AOFAS hindfoot activity scores, as well as SF-36 scores, particularly in the subscales of physical function and mental health. They also found that patients with CCJ incongruity had significantly more difficulty walking on rough surfaces than those without involvement of the CCJ. Importantly, the authors also found no correlation between the quality of reduction of the posterior facet and CCJ reduction, suggesting that CCJ malreduction or nonreduction may lead to more functional limitation than previously thought.

Overall, there continues to remain a paucity of data regarding the impact of unsatisfactory reduction of the CCJ on functional outcomes, and as such the role of the CCJ in transverse tarsal joint mechanics and overall gait kinematics in these patients remains poorly understood. However, as these data suggest, both the calcaneocuboid and talocalcaneal joints play an integral role in the kinematics of subtalar motion and gait mechanics. The CCJ and anterior process additionally comprise a significant portion of the lateral column. Postoperative displacement leading to a shortened anterolateral fragment and shortens the calcaneus. Further studies are needed to more clearly define the impact of the CCJ on outcomes in DIACFs, from both a clinical and a biomechanical standpoint.

Addressing associated pathology: peroneal tendons

Subluxation and dislocation of the peroneal tendons may accompany cases of acute fractures of the calcaneus. These injuries are difficult to diagnose clinically at the time of injury because the pain and edema that go along with the fracture limit physical examination of the tendons.

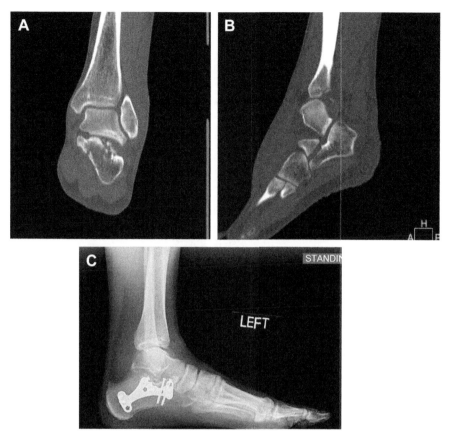

Fig. 3. Sanders type III fracture with comminution of the lateral aspect of the posterior facet (A) and calcaneocuboid joint disruption with a greater than 2 mm articular stepoff (B). Lateral radiograph after open reduction and internal fixation. The large anterior process fracture was reduced first and stabilized with dorsal to plantar partially threaded screws (C).

Although typically used for bony detail in the setting of calcaneal fractures, axial CT scans in the soft tissue algorithm are also helpful in evaluating for peroneal tendon displacement (Fig. 4).

In a retrospective review by Toussaint and colleagues,[50] 421 CT scans were evaluated for evidence of peroneal tendon subluxation or dislocation. Tendon displacement was identified in 118 of the cases (28%). Interestingly, only 12 of the 118 cases of peroneal tendon displacement were noted in the original radiology reports. Factors significantly associated with peroneal displacement included increased heel width and fracture severity (according to the Sanders classification). Joint depression fractures demonstrated peroneal tendon displacement more frequently than tongue-type fractures.

Ketz and colleagues[51] found a similar rate of 47 of 155 (30%) peroneal tendon displacement on evaluation of preoperative CT scan. However, intraoperative examination of the same patients determined that only 18 of the 155 cases (11.6%) had true peroneal subluxation or dislocation. Furthermore, of those 18 cases, just 10 were identified on the preoperative CT scan. Using intraoperative examination as the standard, they determined rates of 56% sensitivity and 79% specificity for CT scan in the identification of peroneal tendon instability.

These authors' preferred surgical technique
Our preference is to use the sinus tarsi approach for all operatively treated fractures of the calcaneus, regardless of severity. The incision begins just posterior to the tip of the fibula and extends toward the base of the fourth metatarsal, ending approximately 1 cm distal to the CCJ (Fig. 5). The peroneal tendons are identified and a small incision is made in the sheath near the tip of the fibula. A freer elevator is passed into the proximal peroneal sheath posterior to the fibula. We then attempt to push the freer elevator onto the lateral border of the fibula to evaluate for rupture of the peroneal retinaculum. If the

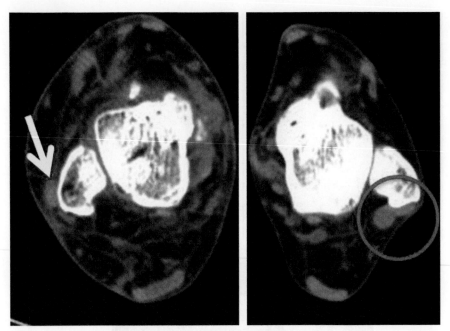

Fig. 4. Axial soft tissue computed tomography images in a 46-year-old male who presented with bilateral calcaneal fractures after a fall off a roof. In the image on the left (right ankle), peroneal tendons are displaced from fibular groove (*yellow arrow*), whereas in the image on the right (left ankle), tendons remain located posterior to the fibula (*red circle*).

freer passes easily onto the lateral border of the fibula, it indicates injury to the peroneal retinaculum. In these cases, the incision is extended proximally to perform retinacular repair.

At this point, the peroneals are retracted plantarward and sharp dissection with a knife or sharp elevator is used to elevate the soft tissues from the lateral wall of the calcaneus. It is easiest to do this while standing on the opposite side of the bed from the usual working position so that the surgeon is able to push the elevator away, rather than pull it toward them.

Next, any remaining lateral capsule of the subtalar joint is incised and the floor of the sinus tarsi is debrided thoroughly to allow for adequate visualization and mobilization of fracture fragments. The lateral wall is pulled laterally to expose the impacted fragments of the posterior facet. In most cases, it is not necessary to remove the lateral wall from the wound completely when using this approach. The posterior tuberosity is mobilized by after the primary fracture line with a blunt elevator through the medial wall of the calcaneus; this allows for later reduction of heel varus.

Once the fracture fragments have been mobilized, the posterior facet is reduced and temporarily stabilized with K-wires. The ideal starting position of the K-wires is a few millimeters below the articular surface to avoid penetration into the joint. The position and length of the K-wires is checked with lateral, Broden's and axial views and then the wires are overdrilled and replaced with 1 or 2 partially threaded, cannulated 3.0 mm screws. Anterior process comminution is reduced and fixed with 3.0 cannulated screws as well. The lateral capsule of the CCJ can be released to visualize the articular reduction.

Once the articular surfaces are reduced, the height and length of the calcaneus are restored. The height is achieved by placing a lamina spreader between the talar neck and sinus tarsi so that the anterior portion of the calcaneus can be pushed downward to correct the angle of Gissane (Fig. 6). A second lamina spreader

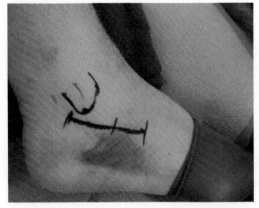

Fig. 5. Authors' preferred incision for the sinus tarsi approach.

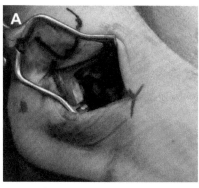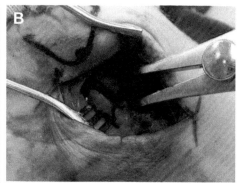

Fig. 6. Exposure of Sanders type II fracture with lateral joint depression (*A*). The posterior facet has been reduced and stabilized with screws; the lamina spreader is between the sinus tarsi floor and talar neck (*B*).

placed into the fractured calcaneus between the posterior facet and posterior tuberosity of the calcaneus is then placed as well to correct length and provide additional height for the posterior facet if necessary. K-wires are then placed from the posterior tuberosity to the anterior process (to maintain length) and from the posterior tuberosity to the subchondral surface of the posterior facet (to maintain height; Fig. 7). The lamina spreaders are removed. Large bony voids may be filled with allograft cancellous chips if desired at this point. The lateral wall is replaced and a sinus tarsi plate is applied. The plate is secured with at least 2 screws to both the anterior process and posterior facet fragments. If the posterior tuberosity has been adequately mobilized and reduced with the placement of the lamina spreaders, a Shantz pin may not be necessary and placement of the posterior tuberosity screws in the plate may pull the heel out of varus. If the posterior tuberosity is not reduced adequately, a Shantz pin is placed through a

stab incision into the posterior tuberosity and used to manipulate it out of varus and equinus so that it may be fixed to the plate. Final radiographs include lateral, Broden's, axial, and foot oblique (to assess reduction of the CCJ) views.

SUMMARY

Displaced intraarticular fractures of the calcaneus continue to represent a technically challenging injury from a management standpoint. Although there is conflicting evidence in the literature regarding the advantages and disadvantages of operative versus nonoperative treatment, there is a growing body of literature to suggest that operative management with near-anatomic reduction of the posterior facet and restoration of overall calcaneal morphology offers greater potential for superior short- and long-term outcomes. These include quicker return to function, greater patient satisfaction, decreased rates of symptomatic subtalar arthritis, and superior outcomes of subtalar arthrodesis in the setting of symptomatic post-traumatic arthritis. A thorough understanding of calcaneal anatomy, fracture pattern, and associated injuries, along with careful selection of surgical approach and timing to surgery, are all critical to minimize the risk of complication and maximize potential for optimal outcomes.

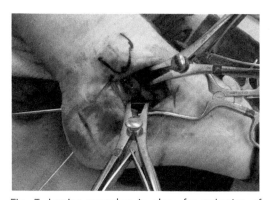

Fig. 7. Lamina spreaders in place for reduction of calcaneal height and length. K-wires are placed percutaneously into the heel for temporary stabilization so that the lamina spreaders can be removed and the plate applied.

REFERENCES

1. Cave EF. Fracture of the os calcis—the problem in general. Clin Orthop Relat Res 1963;30:64–6.
2. Van Tetering EAA, Buckley RE. Functional outcome (SF-36) of patients with displaced calcaneal fractures compared with SF-36 normative data. Foot Ankle Int 2004;25:733–8.
3. Buckley R, Tough S, McCormack R, et al. Operative compared with non-operative treatment of displaced intra-articular calcaneus fractures: a prospective,

randomized, controlled multi-center trial. J Bone Joint Surg Am 2002;84-A(10):1733–44.

4. Agren PH, Wretenberg P, Sayed-Noor AS. Operative versus non-operative treatment of displaced intra-articular calcaneus fractures: a prospective, randomized, controlled multicenter trial. J Bone Joint Surg Am 2013;95(15):1351–7.

5. Ibrahim T, Rowsell M, Rennie W, et al. Displaced intra-articular calcaneal fractures: 15-year follow-up of a randomized controlled trial of conservative versus operative treatment. Injury 2007;38:848–55.

6. Veltman ES, Doornberg JN, Stufkens SAS, et al. Long-term outcomes of 1730 calcaneal fractures: systematic review of the literature. J Foot Ankle Surg 2013;52:486–90.

7. Agren P-H, Mukka S, Tullberg T, et al. Factors affecting long-term treatment results of displaced intra-articular calcaneal fractures: a Post-Hoc analysis of a prospective, randomized, controlled, multi-center trial. J Orthop Trauma 2014;28(10):564–8.

8. Brauer CA, Manns BJ, Ko M, et al. An economic evaluation of operative compare with non-operative management of displaced intra-articular calcaneus fractures. J Bone Joint Surg Am 2005;87-A(12):2741–9.

9. Radnay CS, Clare MP, Sanders RW. Subtalar fusion after displaced intra-articular calcaneal fractures: does initial operative treatment matter? J Bone Joint Surg Am 2009;91-A(3):541–6.

10. Berberian W, Sood A, Karanfilian B, et al. Displacement of the Sustentacular Fragment in Intra-Articular Calcaneal Fractures. J Bone Joint Surg Am 2013;95:995–1000.

11. Gitajn IL, Abousayed M, Toussaint RJ, et al. Anatomic alignment and integrity of the sustentaculum tali in intra-articular calcaneal fractures: is the sustentaculum tali truly constant? J Bone Joint Surg Am 2014;96:1000–5.

12. Stephenson JR. Surgical treatment of displaced intra-articular fractures of the calcaneus. A combined lateral and medial approach. Clin Orthop Relat Res 1993;290:68.

13. Johnson EE, Gebhardt JS. Surgical management of calcaneal fractures using bilateral incisions and minimal internal fixation. Clin Orthop Relat Res 1993;(290):117–24.

14. Zwipp H, Tscherne H, Thermann H, et al. Osteosynthesis of displaced intra-articular fractures of the calcaneus. Results in 123 cases. Clin Orthop Relat Res 1993;(290):76–86.

15. Paley D, Hall H. Calcaneal fractures: can we put humpty-dumpty together again? Orthop Clin North Am 1989;20(4):665–7.

16. Epstein N, Chandran S, Chou L. Current concepts review: intra-articular fractures of the calcaneus. Foot Ankle Int 2012;33(1):79–96.

17. Utukuri MM, Knowles D, Smith KL, et al. The value of the axial view in assessing calcaneal fractures. Injury 2000;31(5):325–6.

18. Csizy M, Buckley R, Tough S, et al. Displaced intra-articular calcaneal fractures: variable predicting late subtalar fusion. J Orthop Trauma 2003;17(2):106–12.

19. Su Y, Chen W, Zhang T, et al. Bohler's angle's role in assessing the injury severity and functional outcome for displaced intra-articular calcaneal fractures: a retrospective study. BMC Surg 2013;13:40.

20. Sanders R. Intra-articular fractures of the calcaneus: present state of the art. J Orthop Trauma 1992;(6):252–65.

21. Sharr PJ, Mangupli MM, Winson IG, et al. Current management options for displaced intra-articular calcaneal fractures: non operative, ORIF, minimally invasive reduction and fixation or primary ORIF and subtalar arthrodesis. A contemporary review. Foot Ankle Surg 2016;22:1–8.

22. Potenza V, Caterini R, Farsetti P, et al. Primary subtalar arthrodesis for the treatment of comminuted intra-articular calcaneal fractures. Injury 2010;41:702–6.

23. Lindsay R, Dewar R. Fractures of the os calcis. Am Surg 1958;95:555–76.

24. Rowe C, Sakellarides H, Freeman P, et al. Fractures of the os calcis. JAMA 1963;184:920–3.

25. Pozo JL, Kirwan RO, Jackson AM. The long-term results of conservative management of severely displaced fractures of the calcaneus. J Bone Joint Surg Br 1984;66:386–90.

26. Hammesfahr JF. Surgical treatment of calcaneal fractures. Orthop Clin North Am 1989;20:679–89.

27. Clare MP, Lee WE, Sanders RW. Intermediate to long-term results of a treatment protocol for calcaneal fracture malunions. J Bone Joint Surg Am 2005;87-A(5):963–73.

28. Sanders R. Current concepts review. Displaced intra-articular fractures of the calcaneus. J Bone Joint Surg Am 2000;82:225–50.

29. Sanders R, Fortin P, DiPasquale T, et al. Operative treatment in 120 displaced intra-articular calcaneal fractures. Results using a prognostic computed tomography scan classification. Clin Orthop Relat Res 1993;290:87–95.

30. Buckley R, Leighton R, Sanders D, et al. Open reduction and internal fixation compared with ORIF and primary subtalar arthrodesis for the treatment of Sanders-Type IV calcaneal fractures: a randomized, multicenter trial. J Orthop Trauma 2014;28(10):577–83.

31. Eastwood DM, Langkamer VD, Atkins RM. Intra-articular fractures of the calcaneum. Part II: open reduction and internal fixation by the extended lateral trans-calcaneal approach. J Bone Joint Surg Br 1993;75:189–95.

32. Schepers T, van Lieshout EMM, van Ginhoven TM, et al. Current concepts in the treatment of intra-articular calcaneal fractures: results of a nationwide survey. Int Orthop 2008;32(5):711–5.

33. Hsu AR, Anderson RB, Cohen BE. Advances in surgical management of intra-articular calcaneus fractures. J Am Acad Orthop Surg 2015;23:399–407.

34. Bergin PF, Psaradellis T, Krosin MT, et al. Inpatient soft tissue protocol and wound complications in calcaneus fractures. Foot Ankle Int 2012;33(6):492–7.

35. Kline A, Anderson RB, Davis WH, et al. Approach for intra-articular calcaneal fractures. Foot Ankle Int 2013;34(6):773–80.

36. Xia S, Lu Y, Wang H, et al. Open reduction and internal fixation with conventional plate via L-shaped lateral approach versus internal fixation with percutaneous plate via a sinus tarsi approach for calcaneal fractures – a randomized controlled trial. Int J Surg 2014;12(5):475–80.

37. Nosewicz T, Knupp M, Barg A, et al. Mini-open sinus tarsi approach with percutaneous screw fixation of displaced calcaneal fractures: a prospective computed tomography study. Foot Ankle Int 2012;33(11):925–33.

38. Zhang T, Su Y, Chen W, et al. Displaced intra-articular calcaneal fractures treated in a minimally invasive fashion: longitudinal approach versus sinus tarsi approach. J Bone Joint Surg Am 2014;96(4):302–9.

39. Kwon J, Guss D, Lin DE, et al. Effect of delay to definitive surgical fixation on wound complications in the treatment of closed intra-articular calcaneus fractures. Foot Ankle Int 2015;36(5):508–17.

40. de Vroome SW, van der Linden FM. Cohort study on the percutaneous treatment of displaced intra-articular fractures of the calcaneus. Foot Ankle Int 2014;35(2):156–62.

41. Stulik J, Stehlik J, Rysavy M, et al. Minimally-invasive treatment of intra-articular fractures of the calcaneus. J Bone Joint Surg Br 2006;88(12):1634–41.

42. Gavlik JM, Rammelt S, Zwipp H. The use of subtalar arthroscopy in open reduction and internal fixation of intra-articular calcaneal fractures. Injury 2002;33(1):63–71.

43. Rammelt S, Amlang M, Barthel S, et al. Percutaneous treatment of less severe intra-articular calcaneus fractures. Clin Orthop Relat Res 2010;468(4):983–90.

44. Woon CY, Chong KW, Yeo W, et al. Subtalar arthroscopy and fluoroscopy in percutaneous fixation of intra-articular calcaneal fractures: the best of both worlds. J Trauma 2011;71(4):917–25.

45. Sivakumar BS, Wong P, Dick CG, et al. Arthroscopic reduction and percutaneous fixation of selected calcaneus fractures: surgical technique and early results. J Orthop Trauma 2014;28(10):569–76.

46. Ebraheim NA, Biyani A, Padanilam T, et al. Calcaneocuboid involvement in calcaneal fractures. Foot Ankle Int 1996;17(9):563–5.

47. Gallino RM, Gray AC, Buckley RE. The outcome of displaced intra-articular calcaneal fractures that involve calcaneocuboid joint. Injury 2009;40:146–9.

48. Kinner B, Schieder S, Muller F, et al. Calcaneocuboid involvement in calcaneal fractures. J Trauma 2010;68(5):1192–9.

49. Forney Hutchinson III, Huebner MK. Treatment of os calcis fractures by open reduction and internal fixation. Foot Ankle Int 1994;15:225–32.

50. Toussaint RJ, Lin D, Ehrlichman LK, et al. Peroneal tendon displacement accompanying intra-articular calcaneus fractures. J Bone Joint Surg Am 2014;96:310–5.

51. Ketz JP, Maceroli M, Shields E, et al. Peroneal tendon instability in intra-articular calcaneus fractures: a retrospective comparative study and a new surgical technique. J Orthop Trauma 2016;30(3):82–7.

Index

Note: Page numbers of article titles are in **bold face.**

Orthop Clin N Am 48 (2017) 105–108
http://dx.doi.org/10.1016/S0030-5898(16)30142-0
0030-5898/17

Moving?

Make sure your subscription moves with you!

To notify us of your new address, find your **Clinics Account Number** (located on your mailing label above your name), and contact customer service at:

Email: journalscustomerservice-usa@elsevier.com

800-654-2452 (subscribers in the U.S. & Canada)
314-447-8871 (subscribers outside of the U.S. & Canada)

Fax number: 314-447-8029

Elsevier Health Sciences Division
Subscription Customer Service
3251 Riverport Lane
Maryland Heights, MO 63043

Printed and bound by CPI Group (UK) Ltd, Croydon, CR0 4YY

08/05/2025

01864696-0011